PRETERM BIRTH

Edited by **Offer Erez**

Preterm Birth
http://dx.doi.org/10.5772/46172
Edited by Offer Erez

Contributors

Erdener Ozer, Anneloes Van Baar, Marjanneke De Jong, Marjolein Verhoeven, Fernando Oliveira Costa, Offer Erez, Saba Masho, Heather Joan Linton Brooks, Michelle McConnell

Published by InTech

Janeza Trdine 9, 51000 Rijeka, Croatia

Publishing Process Manager Ana Pantar
Technical Editor InTech DTP team
Cover InTech Design team

Additional hard copies can be obtained from orders@intechopen.com

Preterm Birth , Edited by Offer Erez
p. cm.
ISBN 978-953-51-0952-5

For EU product safety concerns:
IN TECH d.o.o., Prolaz Marije Krucifikse Kozulić 3, 51000 Rijeka, Croatia,
info@intechopen.com or visit our website at intechopen.com.

Meet the editor

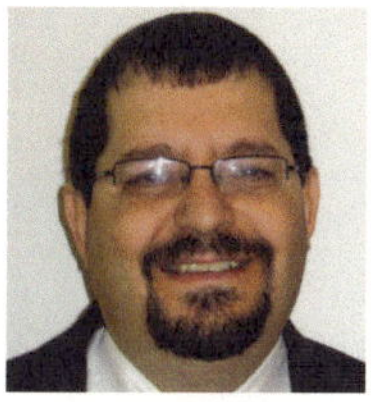

Dr Erez is the acting director of the Maternal Fetal Medicine Unit at the Department of Obstetrics and Gynecology of the Soroka University Medical Center at Ben Gurion University of the Negev, in Beer Sheva Israel. Over the past 16 years Dr Erez has served as a research associate and later as an assistant professor at the Perinatology Research Branch of the NICHD, NIH located at Hutzel Women Hospital and Wayne State University at Detroit Michigan. Dr Erez has published over 140 peer reviewed papers, authored many chapters and served at the editorial board of Peer J and International Journal of Diabetic Research.

Contents

Preface

The preterm parturition syndrome is one of the major obstetrical complications of our time. This syndrome is either spontaneous or indicated, and its prevalence in the USA rose up to 12% of all deliveries. The Institute of Medicine estimated that in 2005 the annual cost of prematurity reached 26.2 billion US dollars.

Preterm labor and delivery has a short and long term effect on the health of the fetus, neonate, child and adult. Preterm neonates are more likely to die within the first year of life and have a higher rate of long term complications including cerebral palsy and autism. Thus, understanding the mechanisms leading to preterm parturition may assist the clinician to tailor the desired treatment that is suitable to the mechanisms leading to prematurity in a specific patient. In the first section of this book we present an update on the association of periodontal disease, maternal stress, and activation of the hemostatic system and preterm parturition. These chapters convey the most updated evidence in each field regarding its contribution to preterm delivery and carry within them the information for further research in these fields. The closing chapter of this section describes the placental pathology associated with preterm birth. Although the results of the histopathological examination of the placenta are often disregarded, it is an important tool in the understanding of the mechanisms leading to preterm delivery. Moreover, since preterm parturition, spontaneous as well as indicated, is a recurrent disease, the results of the placental examination may assist the clinician in preventing the reoccurrence of prematurity in subsequent pregnancies.

The second section of the book deals with short and long term effect of prematurity. Accumulating evidence suggests that the processes leading to preterm birth have an impact on the complications of prematurity. Indeed, chronic maternal infectious morbidity predispose to preterm delivery. Moreover, fetuses who were exposed in-utero to chronic infection or inflammation are at increased risk to develop severe sequel of prematurity including intraventricular hemorrhage, bronchopulmonary dysplasia and necrotizing enterocolitis. This association is eloquently described in the chapter dealing with the connection between inflammation and necrotizing enterocolitis. The second chapter in this section deals with the long term developmental outcome of children following late preterm birth. This is one of the most important topics in modern obstetrics. The rising percentage of preterm deliveries in the past decades is derived mainly from the increase in the rate of late preterm birth. In fact the rate of early preterm birth before 32 weeks of gestation is almost constant. In contrast, there is a sharp increase in late preterm deliveries. The major force that drives the rate of late preterm birth upward is indicated in, some may call it, iatrogenic preterm deliveries. This medical intervention is associated with increased neonatal survival rate and some reduction in maternal morbidity especially due to preeclampsia, obstetrical hemorrhage as placenta previa, and infection associated with preterm PROM. Yet this benefit does not go without a price, indeed, children born between 32-36 weeks of gestation have a higher rate of developmental and school problems than their peers who were born at term. This last chapter brings forward another aspect that is usually overlooked in obstetrical research and that is the long term outcome of perinatal complication.

This book is the second in the InTech series regarding preterm birth and like its predecessor deals with maternal and neonatal aspects of this obstetrical syndrome. Moreover, in this open access series we are able to bring the most update information regarding preterm parturition to the entire medical and scientific community.

Offer Erez
Soroka University Medical Center
Ben Gurion University of the Negev
Beer Sheva, Israel

Section 1

Mechanisms of Preterm Parturition

Chapter 1

Interrelation Between Periodontal Disease and Preterm Birth

Fernando Oliveira Costa,
Alcione Maria Soares Dutra Oliveira and
Luís Otávio Miranda Cota

Additional information is available at the end of the chapter

http://dx.doi.org/10.5772/54977

1. Introduction

Periodontal diseases are chronic infectious diseases that results in the inflammation of the specialized tissues that both surround and support the teeth. It can lead to a progressive loss of connective tissue attachment and alveolar bone. This tissue destruction is characterized by the formation of periodontal pockets that act as reservoirs for bacterial colonization of the dento-gingival environment [1-2]. It is a multi-factorial disease, affecting individuals at different levels of extent and severity. Current concepts on etiology support bacterial infection as the primary cause of periodontal diseases. Periodontal inflammation is initiated and sustained by the presence of dental biofilm, but the host immune defense mechanisms play an important role in the pathogenesis [1,3].

According to the Armitage [3], periodontal diseases can be divided in 2 major categories: a) gingivitis – non-destructive and reversible gingival inflammation related to a non-specific bacterial challenge; and b) periodontitis – destructive inflammation of teeth supporting tissues (periodontal ligament, cementum, and alveolar bone) related to some specific periodontal pathogens [4].

Although bacterial dental biofilms are necessary for disease development, they are not sufficient to produce the disease. A susceptible host is required, and the host response, through release of a broad spectrum of proinflammatory mediators, is responsible for much of the periodontal tissue destruction observed in the disease. Different models of the pathogenesis of periodontal diseases have been proposed [5] pointing to the involvement of cellular and molecular mechanisms of the host and an important participation of neutrophils, cytokines and inflammatory mediators. Therefore, as a chronic inflammatory infectious disease, it can be considered a long-term low-grade systemic stimulus that can affect different parts of the body, a "systemic exposure" potentially harmful to some individuals. Indeed, the association of oral infections and systemic events were present in remote medical records [6]. Mechanisms linking focal oral infections and secondary systemic events can be described as following: a) metastatic infection - result of the dissemination of infection from the oral cavity through bacteremia; b) metastatic injury – result of the dissemination of bacterial products from oral infections; and c) metastatic inflammation – result of the dissemination of inflammatory mediators and immune complexes [7].

There is emerging evidence that periodontal disease is associated with an increased risk of cardiovascular disease [8,9], poor metabolic control of diabetes mellitus [10], and adverse pregnancy outcomes such as preeclampsia [11,12,13] low birth weight [13,14] and preterm birth [14,15] The existence of a relationship between periodontal disease and some systemic conditions or events and can improve care and attention to systemic health, either as a preventive or therapeutic strategy. Therefore, further clarification about the risk association between periodontal disease and pregnancy complications can bring new opportunities and strategies for the prevention of these complications.

2. Problem statement

The aim this chapter is to explore the putative association between periodontal disease and preterm birth, the underlying mechanisms of this association, as well as the current scientific evidence from different study designs such as cross-sectional, case-control, longitudinal, and intervention studies. In this manner, the text will be divided in sections that will describe the changes that occur in periodontal status of women during pregnancy, the risk factors associated with periodontal disease and preterm birth, the biological plausibility of periodontal infection inducing preterm birth, the surrogate microbiological, immunological and biochemical markers for periodontal status and preterm birth, and data from animal and human studies, as well as a critical analysis of the current scientific evidence, the influence study findings on the current practice of Periodontology and Obstetrics and the implications for future research.

3. Review of literature

3.1. Periodontal diseases

3.1.1. Conceptual aspects

The periodontium, also called attachemnt apparatus, is formed by the supporting tissues of the teeth. It comprises the gingiva, the periodontal ligament, the cementum, and the alveolar bone. The main function of the periodontium is to insert the teeth in the jaws and maintain the integrity of the masticatory mucosal surface of the oral cavity [1].

The term periodontal disease is a generic term used to identify an infectious inflammatory process affecting the tissues around the teeth. Periodontal disease initially starts as gingivitis, which is characterized by inflammation of the gingival marginal portion, a reversible and non-destructive gingival inflammation related to a non-specific bacterial challenge. Edema, erythema, and bleeding are clinical signs of gingivitis. When persistent, it can progress to periodontitis, which are destructive inflammatory changes that affect the supporting tissues of the teeth, leading to loss of periodontal ligament, cementum and and alveolar bone [16,17].

This tissue destruction is characterized by the formation of periodontal pockets that act as reservoirs for bacterial colonization of the dento-gingival environment [18,19]. Current evidence [20,21] demonstrated a specific group of gram negative anaerobic bacteria including *Aggregatibacter Actinomycetemcomitans, Tannerella forsythia, Campylobacter rectus, Fusobacterium nucleatum, Prevotella intermedia, Porphyromonas gingivalis* as the main microorganisms involved in periodontitis process. Hence, periodontitis is considered a specific inflammatory process.

It was demonstrated that bacterial species exist in 5 major complexes in subgingival plaque. The 1rst complex, determined to be the red complex, consists of the tightly related group of *Tannerella forsythia, Porphyromonas gingivalis* and *Treponema denticola*. This complex was related strikingly to clinical measures of periodontal disease, particularly pocket depth and bleeding on probing. The 2nd complex, determined to be the orange complex, consists of a tightly related group including *Fusobacterium nucleatum, Prevotella intermedia, Eubacterium nodatum, Campylobacter rectus* and *Parvimonas micra*. The 3rd complex consists of *Streptococcus sanguis, S. oralis, S. mitis, S. gordonii* and *S. intermedius.* The 4th complex was comprises especially by *Eikenella corrodens* and *Aggregatibacter actinomycetemcomitans* serotype a. The 5th complex consists of *Veillonella parvula* and *Actinomyces odontolyticus.*

Virulence factors of most periodontal pathogens mainly involve enzymes with potential to evade or interfere with host defenses and to disintegrate periodontal tissues. The main periodontal bacteria and respective virulence factors and pathogenic mechanisms are presented in Table 1.

Periodontitis is a multi-factorial disease, affecting individuals at different levels of extent and severity. Current concepts on etiology support bacterial infection as the primary cause of periodontal diseases. Periodontal inflammation is initiated and sustained by the presence of dental biofilm, but the host immune defense mechanisms play an important role in the pathogenesis. For disease development, they are not sufficient to produce the disease. A susceptible host is required, and the host response, through release of a broad spectrum of proinflammatory mediators, is responsible for much of the periodontal tissue destruction observed in the disease. Different models of the pathogenesis of periodontal diseases have been proposed [23] pointing to the involvement of cellular and molecular mechanisms of the host and an important participation of neutrophils, cytokines and inflammatory mediators such as interleukin-1 β (IL-β), interleukin-8 (IL-8), tumor necrosis factor-α (TNF-α), prostaglandin E-2 (PGE-2). Therefore, the inflammatory and immune responses basically modulate homeostasis in the dento-gingival region between changes in bacterial aggression or in host defense mechanisms. This balance may favor the onset or progress of priodontitis. Thus, factors or conditions modifying homeostasis of the host can also modify the extent and course of periodontitis, as well as the response to therapy [5].

Periodontal Pathogens	Virulence factors and pathogenic mechanisms
Aggregatibacter actinomycetemcomitans	leukotoxin, apoptosis induction, cytolethal distending toxin, chaperonin 60, lipopolysaccharide, bone resorption induction, vesicles, fimbriae, actinobacillin, collagenase, immunosuppressive factors
Porphyromonas gingivalis	fimbriae, hemagglutinins, vesicles, Ig and complement proteases, lipopolysaccharide, capsule, antiphagocytic products, proteinases, hemolysins and other hydrolytic activities
Tannerella forsythia	proteolytic enzymes, trypsin-like enzymes, neuraminidase, leucin-rich surface protein, adhesin, bone resorption induction
Prevotella intermedia	hemagglutination and adherence activity, bone loss induction
Fusobacterium nucleatum	invasion of epithelial cell, apoptosis activity
Campylobacter rectus	Leukotoxin, stimulation of gingival fibroblasts to produce IL-6 and IL-8

Table 1. Periodontal Pathogens: Virulence factors and pathogenic mechanisms

Current knowledge regarding the multifactorial etiology of periodontal disease puts the individual as a fundamental component. Based on this view, the role of various diseases and systemic conditions in periodontal diseases has been well recognized. Similarly, periodontal conditions seem to be able to modify the physiological balance of various organs and systems of the host. Because it is a chronic inflammatory infectious disease, periodotitis can be considered a systemic stimulus of low grade and long duration, a "systemic exposure" potentially harmful to some individuals [23].

Regarding the epidemiological aspects, periodontal disease is undoubtedly one of the major health problems regarding prevalence of oral conditions in populations. Studies [3,4] reported prevalence of gingivitis and clinical signs of inflammation around 80% in children and adolescents. Gingivitis is, therefore, the form of periodontal disease most commonly found. Periodontitis is presented as different clinical forms: chronic periodontitis, aggressive periodontitis, and periodontitis as a manifestation of systemic diseases. Chronic periodontitis usually has a course of slow progression, while aggressive periodontitis presents a rapid rate of progression [3]. The study on tea growers in Sri Lanka and demonstrated that 5 to 20% of individuals were affected by rapidly progressive periodontitis [24]. However, the chronic form of the disease is more prevalent and occurred in most adults. Studies among adults in the United States foud prevalence rates of periodontitis ranging from 44% to 64% [4,17].

A number of epidemiological studies conducted during the 70's and 80's showed that periodontitis may be associated with risk factors that predispose and modulate the development of periodontal changes. Evidence from longitudinal studies established genetics, smoking, and certain systemic diseases such as diabetes mellitus, as important risk factors associated with periodontitis [4,17,25].

3.1.2. Changes in periodontal status of women during pregnancy

An increase in the incidence of gingivitis and an exaggerated gingival response to dental biofilm among pregnant women has been extensively reported on in previous literature suggesting that hormonal changes can have varied manifestations in periodontal tissues. Several investigations have been developed to assess the different stages of women's lifes and their relationship with gingival health [26-30].

High plasma levels of estrogen and progesterone during pregnancy can influence periodontal tissues through different mechanisms, such as interference in the subgingival microflora composition [27], the modulation of the maternal immune response, and the stimulation of the production of pro-inflammatory mediators [31].

Lopatin et al. [32] observed an increase in the occurrence of gingivitis during gestation with no alteration in the amount of plaque present as well as in the proportion of anaerobic and aerobic species in the subgingival flora. It has been established that pregnant women have a tendency to develop clear signs of inflammation in the presence of relatively little plaque [33]. In addition, another study [34] observed changes in periodontal clinical parameters, such as bleeding on probing (BOP) and probing depth (PD), and reported an increase in clinical attachment loss (CAL) among pregnant women during gestation.

Studies [35,36] showed that high concentrations of female sex hormones stimulate the production of prostaglandin E2 and may exacerbate the inflammatory response of periodontal tissues. Raber-Durlacher et al. [37] reported a decrease in neutrophil chemotaxis, a depression of cell-mediated immunity and phagocytosis, as well as a reduced response of T-cells, associated with increased levels of ovarian hormones, especially progesterone. Lapp et al. [38] mentioned that high levels of progesterone during pregnancy alter the gingival protective response to bacterial challenge due to decreased production of IL-6.

Current evidence from several intervention studies that implemented procedures of scaling and root palning, as well as control of dental biofilm, during the second trimester of pregnancy showed an improvement in maternal periodontal condition with significant improvement in clinical parameters such as gingival bleeding and probing depth, as well as a worse periodontal status among untreated women during pregnancy. These results suggested a substantial benefit in periodontal status, which can have some impact in reducing potential sources of inflammatory mediators [14,39-43].

In this context, the results of intervention studies reinforce the need for oral health care programs direct towards pregnant women, as a way of maintaining homeostasis of periodontal tissues and controlling of periodontal inflammation.

4. Association between oral infections and systemic conditions

Since the most remote medical scriptures, oral infections have been reported as a cause of systemic diseases. There are documentary reports on this subject in ancient civilizations, in the middle ages, and in modern times. During the twentieth century, four key concepts of pathogenicity were stablished: psychosomatization, autoimmunity, autoinfection, and focal infection.

The theory of focal infection, enacted during the nineteenth and early twentieth centuries, stated that foccus of infection were responsible for the initiation and progression of a wide variety of inflammatory diseases. In Dentistry, a large number of extractions were a result of the popularity of this theory. From the second half of century XX, this type of therapy begins to decline in the face of new scientific evidence, revealing that teeth infections could be treated and maintained without necessarily becoming focal points of infection. Recently, advances in several areas of the sciences have provided a more realistic and appropriate analysis of the importance of focal infection in the oral cavity for the rest of the body [5,6]. The literature has suggested three mechanisms linking focal oral infections and systemic side effects: a) metastatic infection - resulted from the spread of oral infection through bacteremia; b) metastatic injury - resulted from the spread of bacterial products from oral infections; c) metastatic inflammation - resulted from the spread of inflammatory products and immune complexes from oral infections.

According to Gendron et al. [19] focal oral infections can be defined as infections that occur in different regions of the human body caused by microorganisms colonizing the oral cavity or its products. Although this concept is highly controversial, it has gained attention by the scientific community in recent years. This is mainly due to: a) improvements in culture and identification techniques that can reveal oral microorganisms systemically disseminated (3), making the oral cavity as an important reservoir of bacterial species; b) epidemiological evidence showing associations between oral and systemic conditions [43].

Periodontal disease can affect the susceptibility of the host, according to Page [21], in three ways: (a) shared risk factors: factors that put individuals at risk for PD may also put individuals at risk for systemic diseases (examples of risk factors and indicators include: smoking, stress, age, ethinicity, and gender); (b) subgingival biofilms: represent an enormous and continuing bacterial load that demands a constant response of the host, as well as a reservoir of bacteria with ready access to the periodontal tissues and the blood circulation; (c) periodontal sites as a reservoir of inflammation: the periodontium acting as a constant source of proinflammatory cytokines, which can reach the circulation and induce or perpetuate systemic effects.

Evidence of a strong association between periodontitis and systemic diseases brought to light the term periodontal medicine, first suggested by Offenbacher et al. [22], to define the field of periodontics studying these relationships. Because it is a chronic inflammatory disease, PD may be considered a systemic stimulus of low intensity and long duration which represents a potentially deleterious systemic exposure. Consequently, some studies have shown that the DP seem to put the host at greater risk for cardiovascular diseases, stroke, diabetes mellitus, lung infections, as well as adverse pregnancy outcomes such as preterm birth (PTB), low birth weight (LBW), intrauterine growth restriction (IUGR) and preeclampsia (PEC) [8-10,15]. Furthermore, Paquette et al. [44] emphasized the importance of periodontal medicine studies on interventional strategies for risk reduction and prevention of systemic diseases.

Based on biological plausibility, it is believed that periodontitis can contribute to adverse pregnancy outcomes throught bacteremia, where toxins and/or ther products derived from maternal periodontitis can reach the bloodstream and cause injury to the placenta / fetal unit. Furthermore, maternal immune response to periodontal infection activates the release of inflammatory mediators, growth factors, and other potent cytokines that can induce the occurrence of PTB (Figure 1).

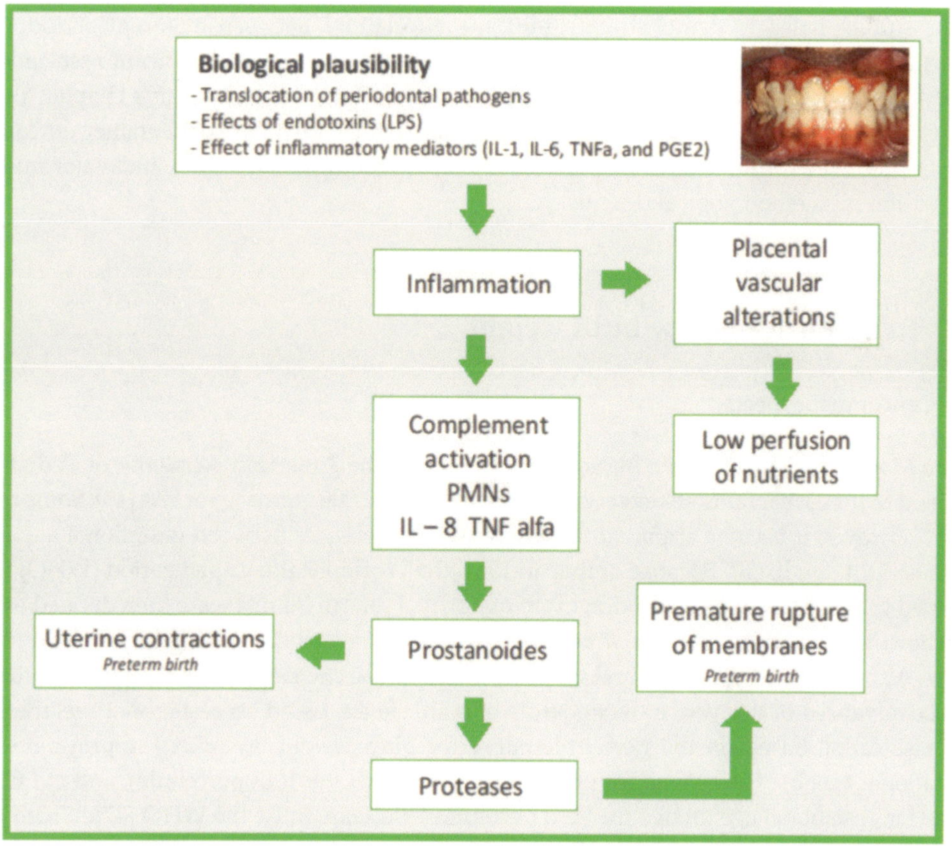

Figure 1. Biological plausibility: association between maternal periodontitis and preterm birth (see attachment).

PTB and LBW represent a major public health problem, ranking among the leading causes of infant mortality. In addition to a great increase in the chance of death during perinatal period, it can result in severe disabilitating disorders, such as neurological problems, lung and respiratory problems, blindness, as well as anomalies and complications due to neonatal intensive care. Preeclampsia, which affects around 10% of pregnant women remains among the most important disorders in obstetrics. It can lead to deterioration of various organs and systems, as well as maternal and fetal death [11,13]. Among pregnancy complications related to periodontitis, intrauterine growth restrictioin (IUGR) can be defined as a decrease in fetal growth observed in at least two medical evaluations at different times which can indicates uterine problems. There are several risk factors associated with the PTB, LBW, and IUGR, including maternal and fetal factors. Special attention should be given to the occurrence of these events in previous gestations. The detection and subsequent study of the relationship between periodontitis and various systemic diseases can improve health care, either as a preventive or interventional therapy. Therefore, further clarification about the risk association between periodontitis and adverse pregnancy outcomes can bring new opportunities and strategies for the prevention of these complications.

Some studies failed to demonstrate significant associations between maternal periodontal infections and adverser pregnancy outcomes, while others showed significant associations with a very wide variation in reported risk estimates. Thus, throughout this chapter, these issues will be critically discussed. A review on the main topic for adverse pregnancy outcomes will be presented considering conceptual aspects, epidemiology, risk factors, and major studies with different methodological designs.

5. Preterm birth and low birth weight

5.1. Conceptual aspects

Since March 1935, after a meeting in Chicago – USA, the American Academy of Pediatrics defined as preterm infants all newborn infants weighing 2,500 grams (g) or less [45]. Some time later, however, it became apparent that there were differences between gestational age and birth weight due IUGR. Because of this, in 1961, the World Health Organization (WHO) [46] defined gestational age as a criterion of prematurity. Preterm infants were then defined as all newborn infants with less than 37 completed weeks of gestation, distinguishing PTB from LBW. Although related, weight and gestational age can be exchange, as well as fetal maturity can be advanced or delayed, independently of both. Hence, based on gestational age, there is a classification based on the percentile curve for birth weight: a) AGA - appropriate for gestational age; b) SGA - small for gestational age (below the 10th percentile), and c) LGA - large for gestational age (above the 90th percentile). Subsequently, the WHO [47]defined the following categories: (a) LBW: less than 2,500 g; (b) very LBW: less than 1,500 g; (c) extreme LBW: less than 1,000 g (d) PTB: less than 37 weeks gestation, (e) extreme PTB: less than 32 weeks gestation; (f) post-term: more than 41 weeks gestation. Since LBW may be a result of

http://dx.doi.org/10.5772/54977

both PTB as IURG, according to Williams et al. [48], it is important to distinguish these two causes when evaluating LBW.

5.2. Epidemiological aspects

PTB is one of the most severe perinatal problems, persisting as a major cause of perinatal morbidity and mortality. PTB and LBW infants represent a major challenge to public health, as well as a social and economic problem, accounting for almost 50% of severe neurological diseases in short and long periods [13,48,49]

The incidence of PTB reported in the literature is varied because it is a multifactorial problem that is influenced by the geographic and socioeconomic factors, racial characteristics, age, and quality of prenatal care offered to pregnant women. According to these authors, PTB occurs in approximately 8-10% of pregnancies in developed countries while in Latin America it may reach 43%. In all populational groups, although a consequence of complexes interactions, birth weight is the most important determinant of the chances of a newborn to survive, grow, and develop healthily [48,50]. Unfortunately, PTB and LBW rates are also high elsewhere: Europe – 4 to 12%, Asia – 15%, Australia – 6%; Africa – 10 to 12%, North America – 7%. Although great advances in prenatal care have occurred, the prevalence of PTB has remained relatively constant over the past 40 years. The inability of health programs to reduce the incidence of PTB is probably due to the fact that the most relevant risk factors have not been well established.

An etiologic classification for PTB was proposed [50], and provided an overview of the key factors for prematurity: a) obstetric causes: primiparity (first birth) in both young and old mothers, small interval during gestations, grand multiparity, previous PTBs, stillbirth previous, multiple gestations, hypertensive disorders of pregnancy, hemolytic diseases, polyhydramnios, low insertion of the placenta, chorioamnionitis, congenital anomalies, male fetal sex, isthmic insufficiency; b) gynecological causes: uterine malformations, uterine adhesions, leiomyomas of the uterus, pregnancy with intrauterine devices; c) extra gynecological causes: socioeconomic and cultural status, malnutrition and anemia, unfavorable profession / occupation, black ethinicity, early maternal age, short maternal stature, low maternal weight, small volume of the maternal heart, smoking, alcohol consumption, hypertensive states, diabetes mellitus, collagen diseases, maternal heart disease, asymptomatic bacteriuria, and urinary tract infection. Considering risk factors, according to Robinson et al. [51], smoking seems to be the main risk factor in developed countries, while poor nutrition and infections seem to be the main risk factors in developing countries.

According to Willians et al. [48], although risk classification systems have been unsuccessful in identifying pregnancies at risk for PTB, some characteristics may be more useful in predicting risk and refer to maternal age, previous PTBs, early cervical dilation, infection of the amniotic fluid, and fetal fibronectin level. One of the best single risk factors in predicting PTB in multiparous women is the previous history of PTB, which can rise up the risk to three times.

However, according to these authors, more than 50% of PTBs are idiopathics. In the studies presented in the next sections, the reported risk estimates presented in the literature for each of these factors will be presented [52].

5.3. Maternal infections and preterm birth and low birth weight

Offenbacher et al. [23] and Gibbs et al. [53], reviewing subclinical infections and PTB, presented the potential biological mechanisms involved in the occurrence of PTB. The authors showed that the translocation of bacterial products and tissue inflammation, with large amounts of cytokines and other inflammatory mediators present in the placenta, are the causal agents capable of inducing changes in fetal development, uterine contractions, and miscarriage. Such mediators, especially, prostaglandin E2 (PGE-2) and interleukin 1β (IL-1β) would be locally produced or transported to the placenta throught the bloodstream. The authors listed the following evidence of the involvement of PGE-2 in labor: (a) the administration of prostaglandins in animal models results in abortion or labor; (2) administration of prostaglandin inhibitors delays the onset of labor delivery and can inhibit PTB; (c) term labor is associated with high concentrations of prostaglandins in the amniotic fluid and maternal serum; (d) concentrations of arachidonic acid, a precursor of prostaglandins, in the amniotic fluid increase during labor; (e) intra-amniotic administration of arachidonic acid in animal models results in labor.

The presence of vaginal infection, even without clinical signs, was associated with the occurrence of PTB, a significant reduction in the frequency of idiopathic PTBs after antibiotic therapy in pregnant women with asymptomatic bacterial vaginosis associated with microorganisms such as *Neisseria gonorrhoeae, Trichomonas vaginalis* and *Mycoplasma hominis* [54]. For Goldenberg [55], genitourinary tract infection is one of the most important factors related to maternal exposure involved in PTB. For this author, this type of infection at any time during pregnancy has the ability to promote the upward migration of bacteria and inflammatory products from the vagina into the coriodecidual space.

Thus, maternal infections may lead to a systemic inflammatory response resulting in inflammation of the fetal-placental unit, including the uterus, chorioamniotic membranes, placenta, and amniotic fluid. This inflammatory stimulus induces a state of activity of uterine smooth muscle by increasing contractility, cervical dilatation, and triggering labor. Infections and inflammation may also induce damage in the placenta, leading to reduced fetal perfusion, IUGR, and fetal distress.

6. Periodontitis as a risk factor for preterm birth and low birth weight

The current concept of pathogenesis of periodonitiss ponts to the involvement of cellular and molecular mechanisms of the host and an important participation of neutrophils, cytokines, and inflammatory mediators such as interleukin-1 β (IL-β), interleukin-8 (IL-8), tumor necrosis factor-α (TNF-α), prostaglandin E-2 (PGE-2) In this manner, periodontitis results in an increase of proinflammatory molecules that can directly or indirectly lead to uterine contractions and cervical dilatation [23]. The presence of untreated periodontitis appears to increase the risk of spontaneous PTBs. However, according to Armitage [56], it is still necessary to determine: a) if periodontal infections increase the risk of adverse pregnancy outcomes in all populational groups accros the world; b) if an cause-effect association can be observed; c) determine the best criterion to characterize maternal "exposure" to periodontal infections. Most studies that evaluated periodontitis as a risk factor for PTB and / or LBW was based on the specific analysis of periodontal clinical parameters. Some studies that combined microbiological and / or immunological factors evaluated the effects of periodontal treatment during gestation on pregnancy outcomes. It should be emphasized that these studies mostly pointed PD as a risk factor for adverse pregnancy outcomes although with varied risk estimates, as previously mentioned.

The first study [23] on the association between periodontitis and adverse pregnancy outcomes was indicated that maternal periodontitis represents a clinically significant risk factor for PTB and LBW. These authors conducted a case-control study with 124 women in the U.S.A. All variables of interest regarding pregnancy, medical history, and characterization of the patients were collected from medical records. Periodontal status was assessed in the postpartum period throught manual periodontal probing with record of probing depth (PD), clinical attachment level (CAL), and bleeding on probing (BOP). The maternal periodontal status was characterized by mean CAL and the extension of periodontitis by the percentage of sites with CAL ≥ 2mm, ≥ 3mm, ≥ 4mm. Cases of PTB and LBW presented worse periodontal status when compared to controls with adequate gestational age and birth weight. Authors demonstrated a high adjusted odds ratio (OR) of 7.9 [95% confidence interval (CI) 1.95 to 28.8] for PTB and LBW in multiparous women and 7.5 (95% CI 1.52 to 41.4) for PTB and LBW in primiparous women. In this study, DP was determined to be an independent risk factor for adverse pregnancy outcomes.

Davenport et al. [57], conducted another case-control study with 800 women from 16 to 44 years from multiethnic groups in London. Women with multiple gestations were excluded from the study. Maternal periodontal status was established by the CPITN (Community Periodontal Index of Treatment Needs) index and general data of interest were collected from medical records. There were no differences between cases and controls in relation to age. A preliminary analysis of data showed a prevalence of CPITN level 4 of 49% in the population, and none of the participants presented CPITN level 0. Authors suggested an association between maternal periodontitis and PTB with an OR greater than 3.0.

Some observational studies found no association between periodontitis and adverse pregnancy outcomes. Davenport et al. [57] evaluated a sample of 236 cases and 507 randonly selected controls, in London. Periodontal examination was conducted with manual probe, and PD, CAL, BOP, and CPITN were recorded. The average age between the case (26.7 years) and control (26.9 years) groups was similar. The factors most strongly associated with PTB and LBW were: hypertension during pregnancy (OR = 3.23, 95% CI 2.05 to 5.10), previous LBW (OR = 2.53, 95% CI 1, 68 to 3.80), smoking (OR = 2.15, 95% CI 1.20 to 3.88). The results showed a tendency that higher maternal education levels were associated with a decreased risk of PTB and LBW (OR = 0.82, 95% CI 0.65 to 1.02). In relation to maternal periodontal status, authors observed that the risk for PTB and LBW decreased with an increase in PD (OR = 0.83, 95% CI 0.68 to 1.00). After adjusting for important factors such as maternal age, ethnicity, educational level, smoking, alcoholism, infections, and hypertension during pregnancy, the risk decreased even more (adjusted OR = 0.78, 95% CI 0.64 to 0, 99). Thus, authors do not believe that strategies to improve maternal periodontal health can be used to optimize pregnancy outcomes.

In Brazil, one study [58] compared three case groups with a control group (n = 393) composed by women who did presented PTB and LBW. Groups with adverse pregnancy outcomes were: LBW (n = 96), PTB (n = 110); PTLBW (n = 63). Clinical periodontal parameters and risk variables were collected for the entire sample. Periodontitis was more severe in control women than in the case group. The extent of periodontitis did not increase the risk for PTB and LBW according to 15 different measurements of periodontitis. Mean PD and CAL ≥ 3mm were also lower in women in the control group.

Lunardelli et al. [59] also conducted a cross-sectional study with 449 women in Brazil, 91.3% were older than 19 years of age and 8.7% were 19 year old or less. The criteria used to define the presence of periodontitis was one or more sites with PD = 3.5 and 4 mm or more sites with PS = 3.5 mm. The controlled variables were age, diabetes, heart disease, socioeconomic status, medical history, genitourinary infection, antenatal care, drugs, smoking, body mass index, and ethnicity. Results showed an OR = 2.7 (95% CI 0.7 to 9.7) for PTB, OR = 2.0 (95% CI 0.8 to 4.8) for LBW, and OR = 1.5 (95% IC 0.5 to 4.4) for PTLBW, suggesting no association between periodontitis and PPT.

Using a different design, a study [60 was conducted in Sri Lanka. Of the total 227 women in the study sample, 66 were diagnosed with periodontitis and 161 were periodontally healthy. The controlled variables were: age, smoking, diabetes, alcohol, socioeconomic status, race, hypertension, previous periodontal treatment, and antenatal care. It was observed an OR = 1.9 (95% CI 0.7 to 4.5) fot PTB and LBW. Authors concluded that the DP was not a significant risk factor for PTB and LBW.

7. Different study designs: association between maternal periodontitis and preterm birth

7.1. Animal studies

Periodontitis induced by subcutaneous injections of periodontopathogens in an animal model (pregnant *hamsters*) lead to an increase in inflammatory mediators levels such as prostaglandin E_2 (PGE_2) and tumoral necrosis factor-α (TNF-α) in the amniotic fluid. Authors found that lipopolissacaryde (LPS) from Porphyromonas gingivalis caused a significant reduction in the weight of the pups, fetal death, and malformations in association with increased levels of TNF and PGE-2. Periodontitis induced by cotton ligature around the upper second molars of adult rats did not promote changes during pregnancy thath resulted in LBW [59].

In the study of Yeo et al. [61], animals in the test group were subcutaneously injected, in the lumbodorsal region, with *Campylobacter rectus*, a pathogen strongly associated with periodontitis. The results showed that infected females presented a greater number of IUGR when compared to females in the control group.

Offenbacher et al. [62] showed that infection induced by Campylobacter rectus lead to structural placental abnormalities and signs of inflammation in the brain, with a 2.8 fold increase in expression of IFN-Y in fetal brain. Birth weight was not affected by exposure to *Campylobacter rectus*, but mortality was 3.9 times higher after a week. However, it was highlighted that the threat of exposure to maternal oral infection during pregnancy can not be limited to the duration of pregnancy, but can also affect perinatal neurological development and growth.

7.2. Prospective studies

Preliminary results of a prospective study [63], comprising a group of 1313 women in the U.S.A, showed an adjusted OR of 4.18 (95% CI 1.41 to 12.42) for women with severe or generalized periodontitis and an adjusted OR of 2.83 (95% CI 1.79 to 4.47) for women with mild to moderate periodontits in relation to PTB and LBW. Two main points were reinforced by the authors: a) periodontitis was present before PTB; b) women with more severe periodontitis had a higher risk for PTB, after adjusting for other known risk factors (smoking, parity, maternal age, and race). Moreover, Romero et al. [64] based on a different parameter, the Russell's Periodontal Index, also observed a decrease in average weight and gestational age of newborns with the increased in the level of periodontitis among 69 Venezuelan women aged between 18 and 35 years. A study [35] monitoring 1224 pregnant women in North Carolina – U.S.A., from the 26th week until delivery and observed an increase in the number of women with four or more sites with CAL $\geq$ 2mm and CAL $\geq$ 3 mm throughout the study and stated that the progressive increase in CAL may be an indication that the activity of periodontitis during pregnancy increases.

Mokeem et al. [65] assessed the prevalence of maternal periodontitis and its association with PTB and LBW in a sample comprising 90 women (30 cases and 60 controls) from singleton pregnancies of Saudi Arabia. The periodontal examination was performed in the postpartum and PD, BOP, and CPITN were recorded. The mean maternal age, socioeconomic status, educational level, history of infection, placental abnormalities, previous pregnancies, prenatal care, type of delivery, and sex of the newborns were similar between case and control groups. Factors associated with PTB and LBW were previous PTB (OR = 4.5, 95% CI 1.44 to 13.99) and previous LBW (OR = 3.76, 95% CI 1.31 to 10, 76). In relation to periodontal status, authors observed in the case group: a) higher mean PD (OR = 12.87, 95% CI 2.27 to 72.95); b) a higher percentage of bleeding sites (OR = 1.05, 95% CI 1.01 to 1.09); c) greater number of sites with calculus (OR = 3.30, 95% CI 1.37 to 8.92); d) higher mean CPITN (OR = 4.21, 95% CI 1.98 to 8.92). Furthermore, it was observed an increased in the prevalence of altered PD in the group of women with newborns of lower weight and lower gestational age, suggesting a strong risk association between maternal periodontitis and these adverse pregnancy outcomes. In 2005, a cross-sectional study [60] in a Brazilian sample of 152 women divided into three groups: periodontally healthy, gingivitis, and periodontitis. Although there was no statistically significant difference in PTB rates between groups, there was difference between birth weight of newborns among healthy women when compared to women with periodontitis over 25 years of age. Therefore, authors concluded that women with periodontitis were more likely to have LBW infants when compared to women with gingivitis and healthy. Siqueira et al. [15] performed a case-control study in Belo Horizonte city, Brazil. The control group consisted of 1042 mothers of term infants and appropriate weight, while the PTB group was composed of 238 mothers of newborns whose gestational age was less than 37 weeks, the LBW group was composed of 235 mothers of newborns weighing less than 2500 g, and the IUGR group was composed of 77 women who had infants with fetal growth restriction. Periodontitis was defined as the presence of at least four teeth with one or more sites with PD = 4mm and CAL = 3mm. Statistical analysis showed an OR of 1.77 (95% CI 1.12 to 2.59) for PTB, OR of 1.67 (95% CI 1.11 to 2.51) for LBW, and OR of 2.06 (95% CI 07 to 4.19) for IUGR. The interaction between periodontitis and adverse pregnancy outcomes presented an OR of 5.94 for PTB, OR of 9.12 for LBW, and OR of 18.90 for IUGR. Authors concluded that maternal periodontal disease was associated with increased risk for these three adverse pregnancy outcomes.

Additionally, a study conducted in Spain [66] to determine the association between periodontitis and the incidence of PTB, LBW and preterm low birth weight (PTL/BW) among 1096 women. The incidence of PT and LBW was 6.6% and 6.0%, respectively. The incidence of the combined events (PTLBW) was lower (3.3%). PTB was associated with maternal age, systemic disease, prenatal care, complications of pregnancy, delivery type, the presence of untreated caries, and periodontitis (OR = 1.77, 95% CI 1.08 to 2.88). LBW was associated with smoking habits, ethnicity, systemic diseases, previous LBW, complications of pregnancy, and delivery type. PTLBW was associated with maternal age, prenatal care, systemic diseases, previous LBW, complications of pregnancy, and type of delivery. Authors pointed the need for further studies since a modest association between periodontitis and PTB was stablished. These considerations also been reported by Agueda et al. [67]. However, another case-control study was conducted in Jordan [68], comprising 148 women who had PTLBW and 438 women with term delivery without vaginal complications, and it was concluded that both the extent and severity of PD was associated with a greater chance of PTLBW.

In 2010, Guimarães et al. [69] conducted another cross-sectional study in Belo Horizonte, Brazil, to evaluate the association between maternal periodontitis and PTB, but also considered extreme PTB. The author's evaluated 1686 women aged 14-46 years and used two different definitions for maternal periodontitis. The fisr definition considered the presence of four or more teeth with one or more sites with PD ≥ 4mm and CAL ≥ 3mm. The second definition considered the presence of at least one site with PD and CAL ≥

4mm. Of the 1686 women examined in the sample, 479 were excluded based on the following criteria: multiple gestations, congenital anomalies, pregnancy from in vitro fertilization, prematurity due to interruption of pregnancy by preeclampsia, heart disease, neuropathy, and placental, uterine or cervical defects. Thus, the control group (G1) was composed by 1046 women with adequate gestation period (≥ 37 weeks), and the PTB group was composed by 146 women with gestation period between 32 and 36 weeks (G2). Another group, composed by 15 women with gestation period < 32 weeks, was determined to be extreme preterm birth (G3). The results showed that periodontitis was associated with a low number of weeks of gestation with OR of 1.83 (95% CI 1.28 to 2.62) and OR of 2.37 (95% CI 1.62 to 3.46) for PTB and extreme preterm birth, respectively.

As previously noted, there were several criteria to define the presence, severity, and extent of periodontitis. The influence of these different definitions on odds ratio (OR) estimates for adverse pregnancy outcomes was very well established in the study by Manau et al. [70], who analyzed 14 definitions of PD and 50 continuous measurements of periodontitis based on 23 previously published scientific articles. The prevalence of periodontitis ranged from 3.2 to 65.9% and OR estimates ranged from 0.62 to 4.46.

7.3. Microbiological and immunological studies

There are also some studies that also monitored microbiological and immunological parameters, or both. In general, most of these studies supported the main clinical findings previously presented. Offenbacher et al. [71] showed biochemical and microbiological evidence that periodontal status of mothers who gave birth to PTLBW infants were significantly worse than mothers of newborns at term and adequate birth weight. The maternal inflammatory response was shown to be an important effector mechanism of the PTB, and maternal periodontitis was an infectious challenge sufficient to result in preterm labor. A complete periodontal examination was conducted in 40 pregnant women and PD, CAL and BOP. The percentage of sites with NIC ≥ 4mm was used as indicator of extension of periodontitis. Samples of gingival crevicular fluid were collected and concentrations of PGE-2 and IL-1β were evaluated by the immunoenzymatic method. Samples of subgingival biofilm were analyzed by DNA probe for identification of periodontal pathogens. The results showed that the case group (25 women) had periodontitis extension index of 42.7% and control group (15 women) had periodontitis extension index of 39.5%. Crevicular levels of IL-1β were increased in the case group, but without statistical significance when compared to the control group. Mothers of LBW and PTB infants showed a two times higher increase of crevicular PGE-2, when compared to controls. Primiparous mothers with higher concentrations of PGE-2 produced the smallest and most premature newborns. Therefore, the authors suggested an inverse relationship between crevicular PGE-2 and gestational age and birth weight, as well as a positive association between these indicators with IUGR. Microbiological analysis showed higher levels of *Tannerella forsythia, Porphyromonas gingivalis, Treponema denticola* and *Aggregatibacter actinomycetencomitans* in the case group.

In a prospective study [72] of 812 women, was tested the hypothesis that systemic dissemination of periodontal pathogens, which could translocate to the fetal-placental unit, are capable of inducing a response of the mother and the fetus leading to PTB. Authors identified *Porphyromonas gingivalis, Tannerella forsythia, Treponema denticola, Campylobacter rectus, Fusobacterium nucleatum, Micromonas micra, Prevotella nigrescens,* and *Prevotella intermedia* in samples of maternal dental plaque and determined serum levels of maternal IgG and fetal levels of IgM to these same pathogens. The results demonstrated: a) a 2.9 times higher prevalence of IgM seropositivity for one or more pathogens among PTB and LBW newborns compared with term newborns; b) the absence of maternal IgG against *Porphyromonas gingivalis, Tannerella forsythia,* and *Treponema denticola* was associated with a high rate of prematurity (OR = 2.2); c) the highest rate of prematurity was associated with low maternal levels of IgG and high levels of fetal IgM. Authors concluded that a direct involvement of the fetus with maternal periodontal microorganisms, as measured by fetal IgM response, provided biological evidence for the association between periodontitis and adverse pregnancy outcomes. They also stressed that maternal immune response appears to protect the fetus from exposure to pathogens and the absence of this protection is associated with systemic dissemination of oral microorganisms, resulting in prematurity.

Dasanayake et al. [73] demonstrated an inverse relationship between levels of maternal immunoglobulin G (IgG) against *Porphyromonas gingivalis* during pregnancy and birth weight, in which the increase of one unit of IgG resulted in a decrease of 5.07g in weight. The authors concluded that maternal serum levels of immunoglobulins against periodontal pathogens during pregnancy can significantly predict LBW. Moreover, elevations in serum level of IL-8 and IL1-β appear to result in premature uterine contractions. Hasegawa et al. [74] evaluated the association of plaque index, gingival index, CAL, PD, and BOP with risk and occurrence of PTB, as well as its association with maternal serum levels of IL-6, IL-8, IL-1β, and tumor necrosis factor-α (TNF-α) in a sample of 88 women. Forty women presented threatened PTB and 18 had PTB. The results showed worse clinical condition with higher levels of IL-8 and IL-1β among women with PPT when compared to those without adverse pregnancy outcomes. Konopka et al. [75] evaluated the association between maternal periodontitis, plasma and gingival crevicular fluid levels of PGE-2 and IL-1β and PTB and LBW in a sample of 128 Polish women. Sample was divided in: a) study group - 84 women (39.2% primigravidae), aged 17-41 years, who had PTB and LBW; b) control group - 44 women (47.7% primigravidae), aged 16-38 years, who gave birth to newborns at term and adequate weight. The periodontal examination was performed by manual probing and assessment of PGE-2 and IL-1β levels in gingival crevicular fluid and plasma by ELISA. The results demonstrated that PTB and LBW were associated with primiparity among women aged over 28 years (OR = 4.0), and with severe or generalized maternal periodontitis (OR = 3.9). In case group, it was also observed gingival crevicular levels of PGE-2 and IL-1β significantly higher.

A recent study [76] was conducted to investigate the presence of *Fusobacterium nucleatum* in chorionic tissues of pregnant women and the effects of this microorganism in chorio-derived human cells. *Fusobacterium nucleatum* was detected in all samples of oral and chorionic tissues of high-risk pregnant women, and it was absent in low-risk pregnant women. It was suggested that *Fusobacterium nucleatum* induces IL-6 and corticotrophin production.

Therefore, some studies reported that the presence of periodontalpathogenic bacteria such as *Porphyromonas gingivalis, Fusobacterium nucleatum* in the amniotic fluid, placenta, and membranes of pregnant women were associated with adverse pregnancy outcomes, including preterm labor and premature rupture of membranes. Findings from the studies by Offenbacher et al. [71] ; Leon et al.,[77] and Gauthier et al., [78] demonstrated the presence of bacteria from dental biofilm in the amniotic fluid and a direct involvment between these bacteria and the fetus. They provided biological evidence of the association between periodontitis and na increased risk for PTB, since amniotic infection is one of the main risk factors for preterm labor [55].

7.4. Intervention studies

Several of the authors previously presented, who conducted cross-sectional and case-control studies, suggested the need for confirming their findings by intervention studies. Some of these studies will be discussed below. Again, despite of some divergences among them, most of these studies support some degree of association between maternal PD and adverse pregnancy outcomes since periodontal therapy in pregnant women appears to reduce the risk for PTB and LBW.

Lopez et al. [79] selected 400 women of low socioeconomic status, between the 9 th and 21 th weeks of gestation, aged 18-35 years, in the program of antenatal care in Chile. The criteria used to define the presence of periodontitis were four or more teeth with one or more sites with PD ≥ 4mm and CAL ≥ 3mm, at the same site. After periodontal examination, participants were randomly divided in two groups: G1 – composed by women who received plaque control, scaling and root planing and periodontal maintenance monthly before 28 weeks gestation; and G2 – composed by women who received periodontal treatment only after delivery. Data analysis was performed in a final sample of 351 mothers who gave birth to live infants, 14 PTB (3.98%) and 8 LBW (2.27%). The G1 group, composed by 163 women, showed 2 PTB (1.10%), 1 LBW (0.55%), and 3 PTLBW (1.63%). The G2, composed by 188 women, showed 12 PTB (6.38%), 7 LBW (3.72%), and 19 PTLBW (10.11%). As in the previous study, the incidence of PTB and LBW was lower in the treated group (1.84%) when compared to the untreated group (10.11%) (OR = 5.49, 95% CI 1.65 to 18, 22). Periodontitis was the most strong factor associated with PTB and LBW (OR = 4.70, 95% CI 1.29 to 17.73) although other factors were also associated with these adverse pregnancy outcomes [previous PTB (OR = 3.98, 95% CI 1.11 to 14.21), less than six prenatal visits (OR = 3.70, 95% CI 1.46 to 9.38), and low maternal weight gain during pregnancy (OR = 3.42, 95% CI 1.16 to 10.03)]. The authors also evaluated whether maternal periodontal health maintenance after the 28th week of gestation reduce the risk for PTB and LBW in a sample of 639 women. The criteria used to define the presence of periodontitis were four or more teeth with one or more sites with PD ≥ 4mm and CAL ≥ 3mm, at the same site. All patients who did not meet the criteria for periodontitis definition or presented BOP in more than 25% of sites were diagnosed with gingivitis or mild periodontitis. A group of 406 women with gingivitis / mild periodontitis received treatment before 28 weeks of gestation. In this manner, they finished the gestational period periodontally healthy and were determined to be the control group - G1. Another group, composed by 233 women diagnosed with periodontitis received treatment after the gestational period, and was determined to be the case group - G2. Authors observed 2.5% of PTB and LBW in G1 and 8.6% in G2. Regarding the association between maternal periodontitis and PTB, authors reported a relative risk (RR) of 3.5 (95% CI 1.3 to 9.2). Maternal periodontitis was the only risk factor significantly associated with LBW, with RR of 3.5% (95% CI 1.06 to 11.4). In the multivariate analysis, the risk factors associated with PTB were: previous PTB (adjusted RR = 4.8), less than six prenatal visits (adjusted RR = 4.7), low maternal weight gain during pregnancy (adjusted RR = 2.6), and maternal periodontitis (adjusted RR = 3.5). Regarding LBW, the risk factors were: previous PTB (adjusted RR = 7.5), less than six prenatal visits (adjusted RR = 7.5), and maternal periodontitis (adjusted RR = 3.6). Authors concluded that maternal periodontitis is a independent risk factor for the PTB and / or LBW.

Evidence from a pilot clinical trial [80], conducted in 366 predominantly african-American pregnant women, showed a PTLBW rate of 8.9% for the group undergoing dental prophylaxis with placebo, 12.5% for women who received scaling and root planing associated with metronidazole, and 4.1% for the women submitted to scaling and root planing with placebo. The OR favoring scalling and root planing with placebo compared to dental prophylaxis with placebo was 0.45 (95% CI 0.2-1.3, p = 0.12). Women in the control group had a rate of 12.7%.

Another intervention study [41] demonstrated that women with untreated periodontitis had a higher risk of PTLBW than pregnant women who were enrolled in a program of plaque control, scaling and root planing, and daily mouthwash with chlorhexidine 0.12% during pregnancy (OR 2.76, 95% CI 1.29-5.88, p = 0.0085).

The results from a pilot intervention study with 67 American women showed that periodontal intervention resulted in significant reduction in incidence of PTLBW (OR = 0.26, 95% CI 0.08-0.85, p = 0.026). Pregnancy without periodontal treatment was associated with a significant increase in PD, plaque índex, and levels of interleukin-6 and interleukin-1β in gingival crevicular fluid [81].

A study [82] evaluated a sample of 450 pregnant women in a prenatal care program in Brazil. Women with risk factors such as systemic alterations (ischemic heart disease, hypertension, tuberculosis, diabetes, cancer, anemia, seizures, psychopathology, urinary tract infection, sexually transmitted diseases, asthma, and human immunodeficiency virus), as well as alcohol, tobacco and other drugs users were excluded from the study. Data related to age, socioeconomic level, race, marital status, number of previous pregnancies, and previous PTB were also evaluated. Initially, the sample was divided in two groups: G1 – with 122 healthy women, and G2 – with 328 women with periodontitis. In G2, 266 women underwent periodontal treatment, but 62 abandoned the study. After delivery, gestational age and birth weight of all infants were recorded and analyzed. The G2 untreated subgroup (n = 62) showed a higher incidence of PTB and LBW (79%). Educational level, previous PTB and maternal PD were significantly associated with current PTB. In this study, maternal PD was also associated with PPT and BNP.

Periodontal treatment was performed on 200 pregnant Indian women diagnosed with periodontitis [83]. The mean gestational age was 33.8 ± 2.8 and 32.7 ± 2.8 in the treatment and control groups, respectively (p <0.006). The mean birth weight was 331.2 ± 2.565.3 in the treatment group and 2.459.6 ± 380.7 in the control group (p <0.006). Authors concluded that periodontal treatment can reduce the risk for PTB in women with periodontitis. Similarly, Radnai et al. [84] concluded that periodontal treatment performed before the 35th week of gestation seems to have a beneficial effect on birth weight and gestational age.

Some intervention studies found no association between periodontitis and adverse pregnancy outcomes. Mitchell-Lewis et al. [39], in a study in the U.S.A, could not associate oral prophylaxis during maternal prenatal care with a reduction in the occurrence of PTB and LBW. A group of 74 pregnant women (G1) received oral prophylaxis during pregnancy, and a group of 90 patients (G2) received no prenatal periodontal care. The prevalence of PTB and LBW was of 16.5% (27 cases) in the sample with no difference in periodontal status between women with PTB and LBW infants and those who gave birth to newborns at term and adequate weight.

Negative results for the association between DP and PTB and LBW were also found in the intervention study conducted by Michalowicz et al. [42]. Randomly selected women received periodontal treatment before 21 weeks of gestation (n = 413) or after delivery (n = 410). Birth outcomes were available for 812 women and periodontal follow-up data for 722, including 75 whose pregnancies ended in less than 37 weeks. Progression of periodontitis was defined as CAL ≥ 3mm. The distribution of gestational age at labor and mean birth weight (3,295 g versus 3,184 g, p = 0.11) did not differ significantly between women with and without progression of periodontitis. Gestational age and birth weight were not associated with changes in the percentage of sites with BOP when compared to study entry.

Oliveira et al. [14] also failed to demonstrate the beneficial effects of periodontal treatment during the second trimester of pregnancy on adverse pregnancy outcomes. In the study, 246 eligible women were randomly divided in two groups: intervention group (122 women with periodontitis undergoing non-surgical periodontal treatment during pregnancy) and controls (124 women without periodontitis with no periodontal treatment during pregnancy). The study used univariate analysis and RR estimates for 225 women. There was no significant difference between groups for the occurrence of PTB, LBW, and PTLBW. RR estimates for PTB, LBW, and PTLBW in the intervention group were 0.915 (95% CI 0.561 to 1.493), 0.735 (95% CI 0.459 to 1.179), and 0.927 (95% CI 0.601 to 1.431), respectively.

7.5. Sistematic reviews and meta-analysis

Finally, it wil be presented evidence from some systematic reviews published on the subject. Madianos et al. [85] selected articles that met the following criteria: (a) assessment of periodontal status by full-mouth evaluation or PD, CAL, and radiographic bone loss evaluation; (b) assessment of birth weight based on weight measured immediately after birth in the delivery room or medical intensive care unit; (c) assessment of gestational age based on the date of last menstrual period or by early ultrasound. Failing to accomplish these assessments, gestational age should be made by the pediatrician through physical examination. The selected studies showed OR estimates for the association between maternal PD and PPT and LBW ranging from 4.4 to 7.9. However, authors concluded that the evidence for this association were still limited.

After a selection of 660 studies by Scannapieco et al. [86], 12 studies met the inclusion criteria. Authors concluded that it is unclear whether maternal PD is a causal factor for adverse pregnancy outcomes. However, authors pointed that preliminary evidence shows that periodontal interventions during pregnancy have a positive impact on pregnancy outcomes.

A meta-analysis developed by Khader and Ta'Ani [87] found that women with periodontal disease had a risk adjusted for the PPT of 4.28 times greater than the risk for individuals with periodontal health (95% CI 2.62-6.99, p <0.005). The adjusted odds ratio for LBW was 5.28 (95% CI 2.21-12.62, p <0.005), whereas the OR for PTLBW was adjusted to 2.30 (95% CI 1.21-4.38, p <0.005). In another meta-analysis [88] the authors reported the RR from intervention studies and found that oral prophylaxis and periodontal treatment could lead to a 57% reduction in the incidence of PTLBW (RR 0.43, 95% CI 0.24-0.78) and a 50% reduction for PPT (RR 0.5, 95% CI 0.20-1.30).

A systematic review was conducted by Vettore et al. [89] on periodontitis and adverse pregnancy outcomes. Among the 964 studies that were first identified, 36 met the inclusion criteria. Twenty-six studies found positive associations between periodontitis and adverse pregnancy outcomes. There was heterogeneity between studies regarding the methods of periodontitis measurement and pregnancy outcomes, which made the conduction of a meta-analysis impossible. Most studies did not control for confounding variables, which makes their conclusions questionable. Furthermore, methodological limitations did not allow conclusions concerning the actual effect of periodontitis on pregnancy outcomes. A possible causal relationship remains unknown. Analytical studies with greater methodological rigor, using reliable measures to assess exposure and outcomes may be important in future research. Polyzos et al. [90] presented the results of a meta-analysis that included randomized clinical trials 7: OR = 0.55 (0.35-0.86) for PTB, 0.48 (0.23-1.00) for LBW, 0.73 (0.41-1.31) for miscarriage / stillbirth. They concluded that the data from the meta-analysis provide evidence for the treatment and enhance the current practice should be evaluated or at least cautious before rejecting periodontal treatment during pregnancy. Meta-analysis by Chambrone et al. [91] from the review of 11 randomized clinical trials identified relative risks of 0.88 (0.72-1.09) for PTB, 0.78 (0.53-1.17) for LBW, and 0.52 (0.08-3.31) for PTLBW. Authors reported that periodontal treatment during pregnancy did not decrease the risk of PTB and LBW. With the goal to investigate whether scaling and root planing conducted in pregnant women with periodontitis reduce the risk for PTB and LBW compared to placebo or no treatment before delivery. Recent meta-analysis [91] analyzed data from 12 randomized clinical trials included in a meta-analysis. The relative risk for PTB was of 0.81 (0.64-1.02). In the group of pregnant women at high risk for PPT relative risk was 0.66 (0.54-0.80). The authors emphasized that there is insufficient evidence to sustain that periodontal treatment during pregnancy reduces the risk for PTB and LBW.

The main studies for the association between maternal periodontitis and PTB and / or LBW are summarized in tables, 2, 3, 4, 5, 6 and 7 according to their methodological design.

Author / year	Study design / location	Sample	Statistical analysis	Outcome / Main findings
Offenbacher et al.[23]	Case-control USA	124 women: 93 cases 31 controls	Logistic Regression	LBW and PTB OR = 7.9 (95% CI 1.52-41.4) (multiparous) OR = 7.5 (95% CI 1.95-28.8) (primiparous)
Davenport et al.[57]	Case-control London	800 women	Descriptive	LBW and PTB OR "/>3
Davenport et al.[92]	Case-control London	743 women: 236 cases 507 controls	Univariate and Multivariate analysis	LBW and PTB Crude OR = 0.83 (95% CI 0.68-1.00) adjusted OR = 0.78 (95% CI 0.63-0.96)
Radnai et al.[93]	Case-control Hungria	85 women 41 cases 44 controls	Logistic regression	PTB Adjusted OR = 5.46 (95% CI 1.72-17.32)
Marin et al.[66]	Cross-sectional Brazil	152 women	Logistic regresion	OR=1.97 (IC 0.4-9.2; p"/>0.05, não significante) Women c/ periodontite maior probabilidade de recém-nascidos com LBW do que com gengivites e saudáveis
Lunardelli et al.[60]	Cross-sectional Brazil	449 women	Logistic regresion	PTB (OR = 2.6, 95% CI 1.0-6.9)
Cruz et al.[94]	Case-control Brazil	302 women: 102 cases 200 controls	Logistic regresion	LBW Adjusted OR = 2.15 (95% CI 1.32-3.48)
Moore et al.[95]	Case-control Inglaterra	154 women: 61 cases 93 controls	Univariate analysis	PTB No association.
Jarjoura et al.[96]	Case-control USA	203 women: 83 cases 120 controls	Logistic regression	PTB Adjusted OR = 2.75 (95% CI 1.01 – 7.54) IgG serum levels and presence of periodontopathogens similar between cases and controls
Moliterno et al.[30]	Case-control Brazil	151 women: 76 cases 75 controls	Logistic regression	LBW Adjulsted OR = 3.48 (95% C 1.17-10.36)

Author / year	Study design / location	Sample	Statistical analysis	Outcome / Main findings
Bosnjak et al. [97]	Case-control Croatia	81 women: 17 cases 64 controls	Logistic regression	PTB Adjusted OR = 8.13 (95% CI 2.73 – 45.9)
Bassani et al.[98]	Case-control Brazil	915 women: 304 cases 611 controls	Conditional logistic regression	Adjusted OR = 0.93 (95% CI 0.63 – 1.41) for LBW Adjusted OR = 0.92 (95% CI 0,54 – 1.57) for LBW an PTB
Siqueira et al. [15]	Case-control Brazil	1206 women 1042 controls 238 PTB 235 LBW	Logistic regresssion	Adjusted OR = 1.77((5% CI 1.12 - 2.59) for PTB Adjusted OR = 1.67 (95% CI 1.11 – 2.51) for LBW
Vettore et al.[58]	Case-control Brazil	LBW (n = 96) PTB (n=110) PTLBW (n= 63) Controls (n=393)	Univariate and multivariate analysis	Extent of periodontitis did not increase the risk for PTB and LBW. Mean probing depth and frequency of sites with CAL ≥3 mm higher among cases
Khader et al.[68]	Case-control Jordan	148 cases 438 controls	Univariate and multivariate analysis	Extent and severity of periodontitis associated with na increased risk for PTLBW
Guimarães et al.[69]	Brazil	1686 women: 1046 controls 146 PTB 15 extrem PTB	Ordinal logistic regression	Adjusted OR = 1.83 (95% CI 1.28-2.62) for PTB Adjusted OR = 2.37 (95% CI 1.62-3.46) for extreme PTB
Nabet et al.[99]	Case-control France	1108 cases 1044 controls	Logistic regression	PTB Adjusted OR = 2.46 (95% CI 1.58-3.83) for PTB induced by preeclampsia

Table 2. Cross-sectional and case control studies

Author / year	Main findings
Collins et al.[100]	Subcutaneous injection of *Porphyromonas gingivalis* lead to a decrease in birth weight, malformation and fetus death in association with increase levels of TNFα and PGE_2.
Galvão et al.[101]	Periodontitis did not affect birth weight
Yeo et al.[61]	Subcutaneous injection of *Campylobacter rectus* lead to a higher occurrence of IUGR
Offenbacher et al. [62]	Subcutaneous injection of *Campylobacter rectus* induced placental abnormalities and brain inflammation but did not affect birth weight

Table 3. Animal studies

http://dx.doi.org/10.5772/54977

Author / year	Study design / location	Sample	Statistical analysis	Outcome / Main findings
Jeffcoat et al.[63]	Longitudinal EUA	1313 women	Univariate and multivariate analysis	PTB OR = 2.83 (95%CI 1.79-4.47) for slight periodontitis OR = 4.18 (95% CI 1.41-12.42) for severe periodontitis
Offenbacher et al.[59]	Longitudinal EUA	812 women	GLM least squares method	Higher prevalence and severity of periodontitis associated with PTB and LBW
Rajapakse et al.[102]	Longitudinal Sri Lanka	227 women: 66 exposed 161 non-exposed	Logistic regression	LBW and PTB OR =1.9 (95% CI 0.7-5.4)
Sharma et al. [103]	Longitudinal Fiji Islands	670 women	Logistic regression	Higher prevalence of severe periodontitis among women wit PTB and LBW (p=0.0001)
Agueda et al.[67]	Longitudinal Spain	1106 women	Logistic regression	PTB OR =1.77 (95% CI 1.08-2.88) No association for LBW and PTLBW
Pitiphat et al. [104]	Longitudinal USA	1635 women	Logistic regression	PTB OR = 1.74 (95% CI 0.65-4.66)

Table 4. Prospective studies

Author / year	Main findings
Offenbacher et al.[71]	Higher frequency of periodontopathogens among PTB with no significance Gingival crevicular fluid PGE_2 levels significativamently higher among women with PTB
Madianos et al. [72]	2.9 times higher prevalence of IgM seropositivity for one or more pathogens among PTB and LBW compared with term newborns Absence of maternal IgG against *Porphyromonas gingivalis*, *Tannerella forsythia*, and *Treponema denticola* was associated with a high rate of prematurity (OR = 2.2) The highest rate of prematurity was associated with low maternal levels of IgG and high levels of fetal IgM.
Dasanayake et al.[73]	Higher IgG serum levels for against *Porphyromonas gingivalis* among PTB
Mitchell-Lewis et al. [39]	Higher levels of *Bacteróides forsytus* and *Campylobacter rectus* among PTB
Konopla et al.[105]	Gingival and plasma levels of PGE2 and IL-1β of women with periodontitis were associated with PTB and LBW
Hasegawa et al.[74]	Worse clinical condition with higher levels of IL-8 and IL-1β among women with PTB when to compared to those without adverse pregnancy outcomes

Author / year	Main findings
Dörtbudak .et al[106]	Periodontopathogens were detected in 100% of PTB cases and in 18% of term birth
Jarjoura et al.[96]	No microbiological differences between PTB and term birth Women with PTB presented higher levels of IL-6 and PGE_2
Lin et al.[107]	Higher pathogens levels and IgG reponse increased the risk for PTB

Table 5. Microbiological and immunological studies

Author / year	Location	Sample	Statistical analysis	Outcome / Main findings
Mitchell-Lewis et al. [39]	USA	164 women	Descriptive analysis Chi-squared test	PTLBW Non-treated group = 18.9% Treated group = 13.5% (p=0.36)
Lopez et al. [79]	Chile	400 women	Logistic regression	PTLBW OR = 4.70; p=0.018)
Jeffcoat et al.[63]	USA	366 women	Intention-to-treat	PTB OR = 0.45 in favor to scalling and root planing when compared to dental prophylaxis (p= 0.12)
López et al. [40]	Chile	870 women	Logistic regression	PTB and LBW OR = 2.76 (95% CI 1.29-5.88, p=0.008)
Offenbacher et al. [59]	USA	67 women	Logistic regression ANCOVA	Treatment decrease the OR for PTB OR = 0.26 (95 CI 0.08-0.85)
Michalowicz et al. [43]	USA	823 women	Hazard ratio Intention-to-treat	Progression of periodontitis were not associated with PTB and LBW RR = 0.93 (95% CI 0.63-1.37) for PTB
Sadatmansouri et al. [108]	Iran	30 women	Intention-to-treat analysis	Periodontal treatment reduced the incidence of PTB
Gazolla et al.[82]	Brazil	450 women	Univariate analysis	Non-treated group presented a higher incidence of PTB and LBW
Tarannum and Faizuddin[83]	India	200 women	Intention-to-treat analysis Multiple regression model	Treatment reduced the risk for PTB
Newnham et al.[109]	Australia	1087 women	Odds ratio (adjusted) Intention-to-treat analysis	PTB OR = 1.05 (95% CI 0.7-1.58)

Author / year	Location	Sample	Statistical analysis	Outcome / Main findings
Offenbacher et al. [81]	USA	1020 pregman women	Chi-squared test	Incidence of PTB was 11.2% among periodontally healthy women, compared with 28.6% in women with moderate-severe periodontal disease (RR= 1.6; CI: 1.1-2.3).
Radnai et al.[84]	Hungria	83 women	Logistic regression	Periodontl treatment showed beneficial effects
Oliveira et al.[14]	Brazil	246 women	Univariate analysis Relative risk	Treatment did not reduced the risk for PTB and LBW
Deppe et al.[110]	Germany	Treated group = 302 Non-treated group = 14 28 with no need for treatment	Chi-squared test	Full-mouth periodontal treatment did not reduced the incedence of PTB and LBW

Table 6. Intervention studies

Author / year	Studies	Main findings
Madianos et al. [85]	Cross-sectional, case-control and cohort studies	Limited evidence is avaiable
Scannapieco et al.[86]	12 cross-sectional studies and rondomized clinical trials	The association is not well established. Periodontal treatment during gestation may reduce PTB and LBW
Khader and Ta'ani et al.[87]	5 cross-sectional and case-control studies and rondomized clinical trials	Adjusted OR = 4.28 (95% CI 2.62-6.99) for PTB Adjusted OR = 5.28 (95% CI 2.21-12.62) for LBW Adjusted OR = 2.30 (95% CI 1.21-4.38) for PTLBW Periodontitis significantly increase the risk for PTB and LBW
Xiong et al.[88]	26 case-control studies 13 cohort studies (Sistematic review) 5 clinical trials (Meta-analysis)	29 studies showed a significant association 15 studies showed no association There is no sufficient evidence that periodontl treatment reduced the risk for PTB and LBW RR = 0.53 (95% CI 0.30-0.95) for PTLBW RR = 0.79 (95% CI 0.55-1.11) for PTB RR = 0.86 (95% CI 0.58-1.29) for LBW

Author / year	Studies	Main findings
Vettore et al.[89]	36 case-control and cohort studies and rondomized clinical trials	26 showed a significant association for PTLBW There is no sufficient evidence about the risk of periodontitis for PTB and LBW
Vergnes and Sixou[111]	17 observational studies	OR = 2.83 (95% CI 1.95-4.10) for PTB and LBW
Polyzos et al. [90]	7 rondomized clinial trials (Meta-analysis)	OR = 0.55 (95% CI 0.35-0.86) for PTB OR = 0.48 (95% CI 0.23-1.00) for LBW OR = 0.73 (95% CI 0.41-1.31) aborto/ natimorto. Caution should be exercized when rejecting periodontal treatment during gestation
Chambrone et al.[91]	11 rondomized clinial trials (Meta-analysis)	RR = 0.88 (95% CI 0.72-1.09) for PTB OR = 0.78 (95% CI 0.53-1.17) for LBW OR = 0.52 (95% CI 0.08-3.31) for PTLBW Periodontal treatment did not reduced the risk for PTB and LBW
Kim et al.[112]	12 rondomized clinial trials (Meta-analysis)	RR = 0.81 (95% CI 0.64-1.02) for PTB RR = 0.66 (95% CI 0.54-0.80) for higher risk group of PTB There is no sufficient evidence that periodontal treatment reduced the risk for PTB and LBW

Table 7. Sistematic reviews and meta-analysis

8. Conclusions

Studies on the association betweem periodontitis and adverse pregnancy outcomes began in 1996 when Offenbacher et al. [5] demonstrated a strong association between these two conditions. Results from this first study called the attention of the scientific community mainly because of the impressive OR of 7.9 for pregnant women with periodontitis having PPT and LBW. Since then, several studies and reviews have been conducted on this topic. However, as noted in this review, conflicting findings have been reported, since a large number of observational, cross-sectional, and case-control studies showed a positive association, while others failed to demonstrate such association. Moreover, there ais a small number of intervention studies and the available meta-analysis also revealed contradictory results. Therefore, current knowledge about the potential association between periodontal infection and adverse pregnancy outcomes is inconclusive.

Divergence in the results of most studies is in great part due to methodological diversity. Some studies also present some deficiencies, such as small sample size, limited and insufficient statistical analysis, inadequate assessment of gestational age and parameters used for periodontitis definition. Additionally, it is very common an inadequate control for potential confounders, with an inconsistency in the control of other variables such as psychological stress, physical activity, weight gain during pregnancy, violence, economic status, and social support. These issues are not sufficiently studied and therefore give rise to doubts about the conclusions of many of these studies.

9. Future research implications

In this sense, it is important to conduct studies with greater methodological rigor, especially those with prospective and intervention design, directed towards looking for information on the effect of pregnancy on clinical periodontal condition and to validate the possible association between periodontal infection and adverse pregnancy outcomes. The study of clinical response to periodontal treatment can enhance the benefits of treatment in the oral health of pregnant women, reducing inflammatory mediators and minimizing the potential impact of periodontal disease on gestation length and birth weight.

The existence of a bidirectional relationship between various systemic diseases and periodontal disease can improve care and attention to systemic health, either in a preventive or thereutic strategy. Thus, a greater clarification of the risk relationships between periodontal disease and pregnancy complications can bring new opportunities the research and strategies for the prevention of these complications.

Abbreviations

Bleeding on probing (BOP)

Clinical attachment loss (CAL)

Confidence intervals (CI)

Community Periodontal Index of Treatment Needs (CPITN)

Interleukin-1 β (IL-β)

Interleukin-8 (IL-8)

Intrauterine growth restriction (IUGR)

Low birth weight (LBW)

Odds ratio (OR)

Probing depth (PD),

Prostaglandin E-2 (PGE-2)

Preeclampsia (PEC)

Preterm birth (PTB)

Preterm low birth weight (PTLBW)

Relative risk (RR)

Tumor necrosis factor-α (TNF-α)

United States of America (USA)

World Health Organization (WHO)

Acknowledgements

This study was supported by grants from the Research Support Foundation of Minas Gerais (Belo Horizonte, Brazil) and National Research Council (CNPq/Brazil).

Author details

Fernando Oliveira Costa[2*], Alcione Maria Soares Dutra Oliveira[1] and Luís Otávio Miranda Cota[2]

*Address all correspondence to: focperio@uol.com.br

1 Department of Periodontology, Faculty of Dentistry, Pontific Catholic University of Minas Gerais and Federal University of Minas Gerais, Brazil.

2 Departament of Periodontology, Faculty of Dentistry, Federal University of Minas Gerais, Belo Horizonte, Brazil

References

[1] Flemmig, T F. Periodontitis. Annals of Periodontology 1999; 4(1):32-37.

[2] Shub A, Swain Jr, Newnham JP. Periodontal disease and adverse pregnancy outcomes. Journal of Maternal Fetal Neonatal Medicine. 2006 19(9):521-528.

[3] Armitage, G C. Periodontal diseases: diagnosis. Annals of Periodontology 1996; 1(1): 37-195.

[4] Albandar, JM, Rams, T E. Global epidemiology of periodontal disease: an overview. Periodontology 2000; 2002 29:7-10.

[5] Offenbacher, S. Periodontal diseases: pathogenesis. Annals of Periodontology 1996, 4(1)821-878.

[6] O'Reilly PG, Claffey NM. A history of oral sepsis as a cause of disease. Periodontology 2000; 2000 23:13-18.

[7] Azuma, M. Fundamental mechanisms of host immune responses to infection. Journal of Periodontal Research 2006; 41(5):361-373.

[8] Tonetti, MS. Periodontitis and risk for atherosclerosis: an update on intervention trials. Journal of Clinical Periodontology 2009;36(supp.10):15-19.

[9] Friedewald VE, Kornman KS, Beck JD, Genco R, Goldfine A, Libby P, Offenbacher S, et al. The American Journal of Cardiology and Journal of Periodontology Editors' Consensus: Periodontitis and Atherosclerotic Cardiovascular Disease. Journal of Periodontology 2009;80(7):1021-1032.

[10] Chávarry NGM, Vettore MV, Sansone C, Sheiham, A. The relationship between diabetes mellitus and destructive disease: a meta-analysis. Oral Health and Preventive Dentistry 2009 7:107-127.

[11] Cota, LOM, Guimarães, AN, Costa JE, Lorentz TCM, Costa, FO. Association between maternal periodontitis and an increased risk of preeclampsia. Journal of Periodontology 2006 77(12):2063-2069.

[12] Boggess KA, Beck JD, Murtha AP, Moss K, Offenbacher, S. Maternal periodontal disease in early pregnancy and risk for a small-for-gestational-age infant. American Journal of Obstetric and Gynecology, 2006; 194:1316-1322.

[13] Siqueira FM, Cota LOM, Costa JE, Haddad JP, Lana AM, Costa FO. Maternal periodontitis as a potential risk variable for preeclampsia: a case-control study. Journal of Periodontology 2008; 79(2):207-215.

[14] Oliveira AMSD, Oliveira PAD, Cota LOM, Magalhães CS, Moreira AN, Costa FO. Periodontal therapy and risk for adverse pregnancy outomes Clincal Oral Investigations 15(5):609-615.

[15] Siqueira, FM, Cota LO, Costa JE, Haddad JP, Lana AM, Costa FO. Intrauterine growth restriction, low birth weight, and preterm birth: adverse pregnancy outcomes and their association with maternal periodontitis. Journal of Periodontology 2007 78(12):2266-2276.

[16] McClanahan SF, Bartizek RD, Biesbrock AR.Indentification and consequences of distinct Löe-Silness gingival index examiner styles for the clinical assessment of gingivitis.Journal of Periodontology 2001;72(3):383-92.

[17] American Academy of Periodontology. Position Paper. Epidemiology of periodontal diseases. Journal of Periodontology 2005;76:1406-1419.

[18] Li, X, Kolltveit KM, Tronstad L, Olsen I. Systemic diseases caused by oral infection. Clinical Microbiology Reviews 2000; 13:547-558.

[19] Gendron R, Grenier D, Maheu-Robert LF. The oral cavity as a reservoir of bacterial pathogens for focal infections. Microbes and Infection 2000; 8:897-906.

[20] Cortelli JR, Aquino DR, Cortelli SC, Fernandes CB, de Carvalho-Filho J, Franco GC, et al. Etiological analysis of initial colonization of periodontal pathogens in oral cavity. Journal of Clinical Microbiology 2008;46:1322-1329.

[21] Page RC. The pathobiology of periodontal diseases may affect systemic diseases: inversion of paradigm. Annals of Periodontology 1998; 3(1):108-120.

[22] Socransky SS, Haffajee AD, Cugini MA, Smith C, Kent RL Jr. Microbial complexes in subgingival plaque. Journal of Clinical Periodontology 1998;25:134-144.

[23] Offenbacher S, Katz V, Fertik G, Collins J, Boyd D, Maynor G, Mckaig R, Beck, J. Periodontal infection as a possible risk factor for preterm low birth weight. Journal of Periodontology 1996; 67:1103-1113.

[24] Löe H, Anerud A, Boysen H, Morrison E.Natural history of periodontal disease in man. Rapid, moderate and no loss of attachment in Sri Lankan laborers 14 to 46 years of age. Journal of Clinical Periodontology. 1986;13(5):431-45.

[25] Linden GJ, Mullally BH. Cigarette smoking and periodontal destruction in young adults. Journal of Periodontology 1994;65(7):718-723.

[26] Silness J, Löe H. Periodontal disease in pregnancy. II. Correlation between oral hygiene and periodontal condition. Acta Odontol Scan 1964;22:121-135.

[27] Jensen J, Liljemark W, Bloomquist C. The effect of female sex hormones on subgingival plaque. Journal of Periodontology 1981;52:599-602.

[28] Mariotti A. Dental plaque-induced gingival diseases. Annals of Periodontology 1999;4(1):7-17.

[29] Kornman KS, Loesche WJ. The subgingival microbial flora during pregnancy. Journal of Periodontal Research 1980;15:111-122.

[30] Moliterno LFM, Monteiro B, Figueiredo CMS, Fischer RG. Association between periodontitis and low birth weight: a case-control study. Journal of Clinical Periodontology 2005; 32:886-890.

[31] Sooriyamoorthy M, Gower, DB. Hormonal influences on gingival tissue: relationship to periodontal disease. Journal of Clinical Periodontology 1989;16(4):201-208.

[32] Lopatin DE, Kornman KS, Loesche WJ. Modulation of immunoreactivity to periodontal disease-associated microorganisms during pregnancy. Infection and Immunity 1980;28(3):713-8.

[33] Mariotti A. Dental plaque-induced gingival diseases. Annals of Periodontology 1999;4(1):7-17.

[34] Lieff S, Boggess KA, Murtha AP, Jared H, Madianos PN, Moss K, Beck J, Offenbacher S. The oral conditions and pregnancy study: periodontal status of a cohort of pregnant women. Journal of Periodontology 2004; 75: 116-126.

[35] El-Attar TMA. Prostaglandin E2 in human gingiva in health and disease and its stimulation by female sex steroids. Prostaglandins, 1976; 2:331.

[36] Ojanotko-Harri A, Harri M-P, Hurtia H, Sewón I. Altered tissue metabolism of progesterone in pregnancy gingivitis and granuloma. Journal of Clinical Periodontology 1991; 18:262-6.

[37] Raber-Durlacher JE, Leene W, Palmer-Bouva CCR, Raber J, Abraham-Inpijin I. Experimental gingivitis during pregnancy and pos-partum: immunohistochemical aspects. Journal of Periodontology 1993; 64:211-218.

[38] Lapp CA, Thomas ME, Lewis JB. Modulation by progesterone of interleukin-6 production by gingival fibroblasts. Journal of Periodontology 1995; 66:279-84.

[39] Mitchell-Lewis D, Engebretson SP, Chen J, Lamster IB, Papapanou PN. Periodontal infections and pre-term birth: early findings from a cohort of young minority women in New York. European Journal of Oral Science 2001; 109:34-39.

[40] López NJ, Smith PC, Gutierrez J. Periodontal therapy may reduce the risk of preterm low birth weight in women with periodontal disease: a randomized controlled trial. Journal of Periodontology 2002; 73:911-924.

[41] López NJ, Da Silva I, Ipinza J, Gutierrez J. Periodontal therapy reduces the rate of preterm low birth weight in women with pregnancy-associated gingivitis. Journal of Periodontology 2005; 76:2144-2153.

[42] Michalowicz BS, Hodges JS, Diangelis AJ, Lupo VR, Novak MJ, Ferguson JE et al. Treatment of periodontal disease and the risk of preterm birth. The New England Journal of Medicine 2006; 355:1885-1894.

[43] Michalowicz BS, Hodges JS, Novak MJ, Buchanan W, Diangelis AJ, Papapanou PN, Mitchell DA, Ferguson JE, Lupo VR, Bofill J, Matseoane S. Change in periodontitis during pregnancy and the risk of pre-term birth and low birthweight. Journal of Clinical Periodontology 2009; 36:308-14.

[44] Paquette DW, Madianos P, Offenbacher S, Beck JD, Williams RC. The concept of "risk" and the emerging discipline of periodontal medicine. Journal of Contemporary Dental Practice 1999; 15:1-8.

[45] Julius H, Hess MD. The chicago city-wide plan for the care of premature infants. Journal of American Medical Association 1936; 107:400-404.

[46] World Health Organization. Public health aspects of low birthweight. (In Tech. Rep. no. 217). Author, 1961.

[47] World Health Organization. International classification of diseases. Geneva: Who, v.1 (Revision), 1977.

[48] Williams CECS, Davenport ES, Sterne JAC, Sivapathasundraram V, Fearne JM, Curtis MA. Mechanisms of risk in preterm low-birthweight infants. Periodontology 2000; 23:142-150.

[49] Lopez Bernal A. Overview. Preterm labour: mechanisms and management. BMC Pregnancy Childbirth 2007;1(7 Suppl 1:S2).

[50] Mcparland P, Jones G, Taylor D. Preterm labour and prematurity. Current Obstetrics and Gynaecology 2004; 14:309-319.

[51] Robinson JS, Moore VM, Owens JA, Mcmillen IC. Origins of fetal growth restriction. European Journal of Obstetrics & Gynecology and Reproductive Biology 2000; 92:13-19.

[52] Goldenberg RL, Hauth JC, Andrews WW. Intrauterine infection and preterm delivery. New England Journal of Medicine 2000; 1500-1507.

[53] Gibbs RS, Romero R, Hiller SL, Eschenbach DA, Sweet RL. A review of premature birth and subclinical infection. American Journal of Obstetrics and Gynecology1992; 166:1515-1528.

[54] Mcgregor JA, French JI, Parker R, Draper D, Patterson E, Jones W, et al. prevention of premature birth by screening and treatment for common genital tract infections: results of a prospective controlled evaluation. American Journal of Obstetrics and Gynecology1995; 173:157-167.

[55] Goldenberg RL, Hauth JC, Andrews WW. Intrauterine infection and preterm delivery. The New England Journal of Medicine2000; 1500-1507.

[56] Armitage GC. Periodontal disease and pregnancy: discussion, conclusions and recommendations. Annals of Periodontology 2001; 6(1):189-192.

[57] Davenport ES, Williams CECS, Sterne JAC, Sivapathasundram V, Fearne JM, Curtis Ma. The east London study of maternal chronic periodontal disease and preterm low birth weight infants: study design and prevalence data. Annals of Periodontology 1998; 3(1):213-220.

[58] Vettore MV, Leão AT, Leal Mdo C, Feres M, Sheiham A. The relationship between periodontal disease and preterm low birthweight: clinical and microbiological results. Journal of Periodontal Research 2008; 615-626.

[59] Offenbacher S, Lieff S, Bogges KA, Murtha AP, Madianos PN, Champagne CME, Mckaig RG, Jared Hl, Mauriello SM, Auten Jr. Rl, Herbert WRP, Beck JD. Maternal periodontitis and prematurity: obstetric outcome of prematurity and growth restriction. Annals of Periodontology 2001; 6(1):164-174.

[60] Lunardelli AN, Peres MA. Is there an association between periodontal disease, prematurity and low birth weight? A population-based study. Journal of Clinical Periodontology 2005; 32:938-946.

[61] Yeo A, Smith MA, Lin D, Riché EL, Moore A, Elter J, Offenbacher S.Campylobacter rectus mediates growth restriction in pregnant mice. Journal of Periodontology 2005;76(4):551-7.

[62] Offenbacher S, Riché EL, Barros SP, Bobetsis YA, Lin D, Beck JD. Effects of maternal Campylobacter rectus infection on murine placenta, fetal and neonatal survival, and brain development. Journal of Periodontology 2005;76(11 Suppl):2133-43.

[63] Jeffcoat MK, Hauth JC, Geurs NC, Reddy MS, Cliver SP, Hodgkins PM, Goldenberg RL. Periodontal disease and preterm birth: results of a pilot intervention study. Journal of Periodontology 2003;74(8):1214-8.

[64] Romero BC, Chiquito C, Elejalde LE, Bernardoni CB. Relationship between periodontal disease in pregnant women and the nutritional condition of their newborns. Journal of Periodontology 2002; 73:1177-1183.

[65] Mokeem SA, Molla GN, Al-Jewair TS. The prevalence and relationship between periodontal disease and pre-term low birth weight infants at king khalid university hospital in Riyadh Saudi Arabia. Journal of Contemporary Dental Practice 2004; 5:40-56.

[66] Marin C, Segura-Egea JJ, Martı´Nez-Sahuquillo A, Bullo NP. Correlation between infant birth weight and mother's periodontal status. Journal of Clinical Periodontology 2005; 32:299-304.

[67] Agueda A, Echeverría A, Manau C. Association between periodontitis in pregnancy and preterm or low birth weight: Review of the literature. Medical Oral Patology Oral Cirurgy Bucal 2008; 13:609-15.

[68] Khader Y, Al-Shishani L, Obeidat B, Khassawneh M, Burgan S, Amarin Zo, Alomari M, Alkafajei A. Maternal periodontal status and preterm low birth weight delivery: a case-control study. Archives the Gynecology and Obstetrics 2009; 279:165-169.

[69] Guimarães AN, Silva-Mato A, Miranda Cota LO, Siqueira FM, Costa FO. Maternal periodontal disease and preterm or extreme preterm birth: an ordinal logistic regression analysis. Journal of Periodontology 2010;3:350-358.

[70] Manau C, Echeverria A, Agueda A, Guerrero A, Echeverria JJ. Periodontal disease definition may determine the association between periodontitis and pregnancy outcomes. Journal of Clinical Periodontology 2008; 35:385-97.

[71] Offenbacher S, Jared Hl, O'Reilly PG, Wells SR, Salvi GE, Lawrence HP, Socransky SS, Beck JD. Potencial pathogenic mechanisms of periodontitis-associated pregnancy complications. Annals of Periodontology 1998; 3(1):233-250.

[72] Madianos PN, Lieff S, Murtha AP, Boggess KA, Auten Jr RL, Beck JD, Offenbacher S. Maternal periodontitis and prematurity part II: maternal infection and fetal exposure. Annals of Periodontology 2000; 6(1):175-182.

[73] Dasanayake AP, Boyd D, Madianos PN, Offenbacher S, Hills E. The association between Porphyromonas gingivalis-specific maternal serum IgG and low birth weight. Journal of Periodontology 2001;72:1491-1497.

[74] Hasegawa K, Furuichi Y, Shimotsu A, Nakamura M, Yoshinaga M, Kamimoto M, Hatae M, Maruyama I, Izumi Y. Associations between systemic status, periodontal status, serum cytocine levels, and delivery outcomes in pregnant women with a diagnosis of threatened premature labor. Journal of Periodontology 2003; 74:1764-1770.

[75] Konopka T, Rutkowska M, Hirnle L, Kopec W, Karolewska E. The prostaglandin E2 and inrtelukin 1-Beta in women with periodontal diseases and preterm low-birth-weight. Bull Group International Group for Scientific Research in Stomatology and Odontology 2003; 45:18-28.

[76] Tateishi F, Hasegawa-Nakamura K, Nakamura T, Oogai Y, Komatsuzawa H, Kawamata K, Douchi T, Hatae M, Noguchi K. Detection of Fusobacterium nucleatum in chorionic tissues of high-risk pregnant women. Journal of Clinical Periodontology 2012;39(5):417-24.

[77] Leon, R., Silva, N., Ovalle, A., Chaparro, A., Ahumada, A., Gajardo, M., Martinez, M & Gamonal, J. Detection of *Porphyromonas gingivalis* in the amniotic fluid in pregnant women with a diagnosis of threatened premature labor. Journal of Periodontology 2007; 78: 1249-1255.

[78] Gauthier, S., Tetu, A., Himaya, E., Morand, M., Chandad, F., Rallu, F. & Bujold, E. (2011) The origin of *Fusobacterium nucleatum* involved in intra-amniotic infection and pre-term birth. The journal of Maternal-fetal & Neonatal Medicine 2011; 24: 1329-1332

[79] Lopez NJ, Smith PC, Gutierrez J. Higher risk of preterm birth and low birth weight in women with periodontal disease. Journal of Dental Research 2002; 81:58-63.

[80] Jeffcoat MK, Geurs NC, Reddy MS, Goldenberg Rl, Hauth JC. Current evidence regarding periodontal disease as a risk factor in preterm birth. Annals of Periodontology 2001; 6(1):183-188.

[81] Offenbacher S, Boggess KA, Murtha AP, Jared HL, Lieff S, McKaig RG, Mauriello SM, Moss KL, Beck JD. Progressive periodontal disease and risk of very preterm delivery. Obstetrics and Gynecology 2006; 107(5):1171.

[82] Gazolla CM, Ribeiro A, Moysés MR, Oliveira LA, Pereira LJ, Sallum AW. Evaluation of the incidence of preterm low birth weight in patients undergoing periodontal therapy. Journal of Periodontology 2007; 78:842-848.

[83] Tarannum F, Faizuddin M. Effect of periodontal therapy on pregnancy outcome in women affected by periodontitis. Journal of Periodontology 2007;78(11):2095-103.

[84] Radnai M, Pál A, Novák T, Urbán E, Eller J, Gorzó I. Benefits of periodontal therapy when preterm birth threatens. Journal of Dental Research 2009; 3:280-284.

[85] Madianos PN, Bobetsis GA, Kinane DF. Is periodontitis associated with an increased risk of coronary heart disease and preterm and/or low birth weight births? Journal of Clinical Periodontology 2002; 29 (Suppl 3):22-36.

[86] Scannapieco FA, Bush RB, Paju S. Periodontal disease as a risk factor for adverse pregnancy outcomes: a systematic review. Annals of Periodontology 2003; 8(1):70-78.

[87] Khader YS, Ta'ani Q. Periodontal diseases and the risk of preterm birth and low birth weight: a meta-analysis. Journal of Periodontology. 2005;76(2):161-5.

[88] Xiong X, Buekens P, Fraser WD, Beck J, Offenbacher S. Periodontal disease and adverse pregnancy outcomes: a systematic review. BJOG. 2006;113(2):135-43.

[89] Vettore MV, Lamarca GA, Leão ATT, Thomaz FB, Sheiham A, Leal MC. Periodontal infection and pregnancy outcomes: a systematic review of epidemiological studies. Reports in Public Health 2006; 22:2041-2053.

[90] Polyzos NP, Polyzos IP, Zavos A, Valachis A, Mauri D, Papanikolaou EG, Tzioras S, Weber D, Messinis IE. Obstetric outcomes after treatment of periodontal disease during pregnancy: systematic review and meta-analysis. BMJ. 2010 29;341. doi: 10.1136/bmj.c7017.

[91] Chambrone L, Pannuti CM, Guglielmetti MR, Chambrone LA. Evidence grade associating periodontitis with preterm birth and/or low birth weight: II: a systematic review of randomized trials evaluating the effects of periodontal treatment. Journal of Clinical Periodontology 2011;38(10):902-914.

[92] Davenport ES, Williams CECS, Sterne JAC, Murad S, Sivapathasundram V, Curtis MA. Maternal periodontal disease and preterm low birthweight: case-control study. Journal of Dental Research 2002; 81:313-318.

[93] Radnai M, Gorzó I, Nagy E, Urbán E, Novák T, Pál A. A possible association between preterm birth and early periodontitis. A pilot study. Journal of Clinical Periodontology 2004;31(9):736-41.

[94] Cruz SS, Costa Mda C, Gomes Filho IS, Vianna MI, Santos CT. Maternal periodontal disease as a factor associated with low birth weight. Revista de Saude Publica. 2005;39(5):782-7. Portuguese.

[95] Moore S, Randhawa M, Ide M. A case-control study to investigate an association between adverse pregnancy outcome and periodontal disease. Journal of Clinical Periodontology 2005;32(1):1-5.

[96] Jarjoura K, Devine PC, Perez-Delboy A, Herrera-Abreu M, D'Alton M, Papapanou PN. Markers of periodontal infection and preterm birth. American Journal of Obstetrics and Gynecology 2005;192(2):513-9.

[97] Bosnjak A, Relja T, Vucićević-Boras V, Plasaj H, Plancak D. Pre-term delivery and periodontal disease: a case-control study from Croatia. Journal of Clinical Periodontology 2006;33(10):710-6.

[98] Bassani DG, Olinto MT, Kreiger N. Periodontal disease and perinatal outcomes: a case-control study. Journal of Clinical Periodontology 2007;34(1):31-9.

[99] Nabet C, Lelong N, Colombier ML, Sixou M, Musset AM, Goffinet F, Kaminski M; Epipap Group.Maternal periodontitis and the causes of preterm birth: the case-control Epipap study. Journal of Clinical Periodontology. 2010;37(1):37-45.

[100] Collins JG, Windley HW 3rd, Arnold RR, Offenbacher S. Effects of a Porphyromonas gingivalis infection on inflammatory mediator response and pregnancy outcome in hamsters. Infection and Immunity 1994;62(10):4356-61.

[101] Galvão MP, Rösing CK, Ferreira MB.Effects of ligature-induced periodontitis in pregnant Wistar rats. Brazilian Oral Research [Pesquisa Odontológica Brasileira] 2003;17(1):51-5.

[102] Rajapakse PS, Nagarathne M, Chandrasekra KB Dasanayake AP. Periodontal disease and prematurity among non-smoking Sri Lankan women. Journal of Dental Research 2005; 84:274-277.

[103] Sharma R, Maimanuku LR, Morse Z, Pack AR.Preterm low birth weights associated with periodontal disease in the Fiji Islands. International Dental Journal 2007;57(4): 257-60.

[104] Pitiphat W, Joshipura KJ, Gillman MW, Williams PL, Douglass CW, Rich-Edwards JW. Maternal periodontitis and adverse pregnancy outcomes. Community Dental and Oral Epidemiology 2008;36(1):3-11.

[105] Konopka T, Rutkowska M, Hirnle L, Kopec W, Karolewska E. The secretion of prostaglandin E2 and interleukin 1-beta in women with periodontal diseases and preterm low-birth-weight. Bull Group International Research Science Stomatology and Odontology 2003;45(1):18-28.

[106] Dörtbudak O, Eberhardt R, Ulm M, Persson GR. Periodontitis, a marker of risk in pregnancy for preterm birth. Journal of Clinical Periodontology 2005;32(1):45-52.

[107] Lin D, Moss K, Beck JD, Hefti A, Offenbacher S. Persistently high levels of periodontal pathogens associated with preterm pregnancy outcome. Journal of Periodontology 2007;78(5):833-41.

[108] Sadatmansouri S, Sedighpoor N, Aghaloo M.Effects of periodontal treatment phase I on birth term and birth weight. Indian Society and Pedodontics Preventive Dentistry. 2006;24(1):23-6.

[109] Newnham JP, Newnham IA, Ball CM, Wright M, Pennell CE, Swain J, Doherty DA. Treatment of periodontal disease during pregnancy: a randomized controlled trial. Obstetrics and Gynecology 2009;114(6):1239-48.

[110] Deppe H, Hohlweg-Majert B, Hölzle F, Schneider KT, Wagenpfeil S. Pilot study for periodontal treatment and pregnancy outcome: a clinical prospective study. Quintessence International 2010;41(6):e101-10.

[111] Vergnes JN, Sixou M.Preterm low birth weight and maternal periodontal status: a meta-analysis. American Journal of Obstetrics and Gynecology 2007;196(2):135.e1-7.

[112] Kim AJ, Lo AJ, Pullin DA, Thornton-Johnson DS, Karimbux NY.Scaling and Root Planing Treatment for Periodontitis to Reduce Preterm Birth and Low Birth Weight: A Systematic Review and Meta-Analysis of Randomized Controlled Trials. Journal of Periodontology. 2012 [doi:10.1902/jop.2012.120079]

Chapter 2

Preterm Birth and Stressful Life Events

Susan Cha and Saba W. Masho

Additional information is available at the end of the chapter

http://dx.doi.org/10.5772/54978

1. Introduction

Stress is defined as a physiologic response to psychological and physical demands and threats [1]. That is - when "environmental demands tax or exceed the adaptive capacity of an organism, resulting in psychological and biological changes that may place persons at risk for disease" [2]. Despite the challenges of measuring, defining, and studying stress, a large body of literature documents the contributions of stressors and affective state during pregnancy on birth outcomes [3]. In the last two decades, psychosocial stress has evolved to encompass mental health states and stressors such as anxiety, depression, racism, lack of social support, coping mechanisms, job strain, acculturation stress, and domestic violence [4].

In general stress is divided into acute and chronic stress. While stress may have some benefits in responding to stressors, chronic stress has been shown to be associated with chronic diseases including preterm birth. Acute stress is short-lived, an effective resolution to heightened threats or demands [1]. Examples of acute stresses can be impending final exams for college students, brief relationship arguments, and minor upsets in finances. Chronic stress persists for longer period of time without resolution to threats or demands. Stressors that accompany social racism, prolonged homelessness, living in sub-standard conditions, living in high crime rate neighborhoods, and being a single parent are long-standing and chronic.

Mounting evidence has linked stress to multiple chronic diseases over the years. This is particularly true in studies investigating preterm births. Preterm birth is one of the leading causes of infant mortality and childhood morbidities and it is mainly caused by premature rupture of membrane. Although some of the factors leading to premature births are known, the cause for early labor is not fully understood. In the past decade, the influence of stress on premature birth has received special attention. This chapter discusses the role of stress as it relates to preterm birth. Additionally, the patho-physiologic mechanisms, risk factors, and psychometric measures and biomarkers used to assess stress are examined.

2. Poor birth outcomes and stress

Preterm and low birth weight, and intrauterine growth restriction are the leading causes of neonatal and infant morbidity, mortality, and neurodevelopmental impairments worldwide [5,6]. A preterm birth is the birth of an infant less than 37 weeks of gestation. Preterm birth contributes to other adverse birth outcomes such as low birth weight (defined as 2,500 grams or less), developmental delays, infections and cognitive impairment [7]. An extensive body of research provides evidence for the relationship between stress and poor birth outcomes such as prematurity and low birth weight. Other adverse health sequelae such as birth defects, miscarriages, stillbirth, and maternal complications (i.e. preeclampsia, gestational diabetes, and prenatal hemorrhaging) are also associated with maternal stress [8-11]. Occurring in 8 to 12 percent of all pregnancies worldwide, rates of preterm birth and low birth weight are higher in the United States compared to other industrialized nations [12]. Despite efforts to improve birth outcomes, preterm birth and low birth weight remain a major issue due to increasing disparities in rates [13]. Moreover, certain subgroups are disproportionately affected by the problem. For instance, in the U.S., African-Americans have almost twice the rate of low birth weight and preterm delivery, and three times the rate of very low birth weight (<1,500 grams) and very preterm delivery (<32 weeks) compared to Caucasian Americans [14]. High rates of prematurity and low birth weight are of public health concern because they are the leading causes of infant and neonatal morbidity and mortality [15]. Preterm infants are at higher risk for serious complications such as respiratory, gastrointestinal, nervous system, and immune-related problems [7].

2.1. Preterm birth

The first study to explore the relationship between stress during pregnancy and development biology took place in the 1940's with the advent of Sontag's pioneering work [16]. Sontag observed a relationship between emotional disturbance in pregnant mothers and hyperactive fetuses and early feeding difficulties in their offspring. More than two decades later, Gunter published a report on stressful environmental and psychological factors before and during pregnancy and preterm birth among Afro-American women [17]. Twenty cases of women who experienced preterm birth were matched with 20 women with normal deliveries. Gunter conducted a thorough evaluation using a battery of assessments that included measures of self-concept, psychosomatic and neuropsychiatric symptoms, and life events related to death in the family, desertion, economic need, and physical disabilities. Results implied a relationship between psychosomatic conditions and life or social situation of the mother were related to the outcome of pregnancy. Until the 1990's, many investigations on stress and preterm birth were largely retrospective, riddled with weak conceptualizations and methodological problems that limited conclusions [18]. Since then, the body of research on psychosocial stress and preterm has grown substantially, and though there are conflicting reports, studies have shown that women experiencing high stress are 1.5 to 3 times more likely to experience preterm delivery than less distressed women [7,19,20].

Dole and colleagues conducted a study to examine a comprehensive panel of psychosocial factors among which included negative life events, pregnancy-related anxiety, and other stressors in relation to preterm birth in a prospective cohort study of nearly 2,000 pregnant women in North Carolina [21]. They found that women in the highest negative life events impact quartile had the highest risk of preterm birth (adjusted RR = 1.8, 95% CI = 1.2 to 2.7). Further, pregnancy-related anxiety in mid-pregnancy predicted spontaneous preterm birth even after controlling for a wide range of confounding variables (RR = 2.0, 95% CI = 1.6 to 3.9). There is converging evidence across studies of diverse populations regarding the adverse effects of pregnancy anxiety on preterm birth [3]. Pregnancy anxiety, defined as fears and anxiety related to the health and well-being of the baby, childbirth, and postpartum parenting, predicts the risk of spontaneous preterm birth with consistent results for various racial and ethnic groups [3,22].

Dunkel Schetter and Glynn conducted a systematic review for the relationship between various types of stress and preterm birth [23]. This comprehensive study included more than 80 studies of which most had prospective designs with robust sample size and validated measures. Authors reported that stressful life events, major community-wide disasters, chronic stressors, and pregnancy anxiety increased the risk for preterm birth. Of the studies assessing major life events during pregnancy, more than half reported significant effects on gestational age or preterm birth. Women who experienced stressful life events such as the death of a family member were 1.4 to 1.8 times as likely to have a preterm birth. Similar to other studies, the estimate of effect was stronger when stressful life events took place earlier in the pregnancy. Other types of stress brought on by natural disasters or terrorist attacks, chronic strain (i.e. general, household, homelessness), and neighborhood stressors (such as poverty and crime) also contributed independently to the risk of preterm birth or gestational age. Although studies that used standard scales to measure daily hassles showed no significant effect on birth outcomes, using combinations of perceived stress measures predicted preterm birth in some studies [15,24,25].

Two main factors have emerged as central in better understanding the impact of life event stressors on preterm birth: timing of stressor and self-perceived stress [26]. Several studies have shown a decline in psychological and physiological stress response in pregnant women as pregnancy progresses [27-30]. A paper published in 2001 by Glynn and colleagues reported that women who lived through the Northridge earthquake in California showed a differential response to the psychological effect of the earthquake depending on their gestational age at the time of the event [28]. There was a significant association between women who experienced the stress early in the pregnancy and shorter gestational age at delivery. Participants in the first trimester also evaluated the earthquake as more upsetting and aversive than women in the second or third trimester scoring higher on a life events inventory. Similar results were observed among women who lived through the aftermaths of the terrorist attacks at the World Trade Center on September 11, 2001 [31]. Women who were in their first trimester at the time of the stressful incident showed shorter gestational times than controls; however no difference was observed among women in the second trimester. Considering the time frame of maternal exposure to stress and self-perceived severity of stress may be important in understanding how women's response to stress has an impact on fetal development.

2.2. Low birth weight

Chronic stressors are robust predictors of low birth weight, infant weighing less than 2,500 grams at birth [32]. Although a significant proportion of low birth weight infants are preterm births, several studies have reported the impact of stress on low birth weight. A recent population-based cohort study conducted by Brown et al. sought to examine the social determinants of low birth weight in Australia [20]. One in six women reported three or more stressful life events or social health issues in the 12 months preceding the last birth. Women coping with multiple life events remained significantly more likely to have a low birth weight infant after adjusting for smoking, number of prenatal visits, and other known covariates. Specifically, women reporting three or more stressful events or social health issues had a twofold increase in odds of having a low birth weight infant compared to women reporting no issues. In a U.S. study, maternal stress was associated with 2 to 3.8 times the risk of low birth weight among a sample of nearly 1,400 pregnant low-income women [33]. In fact, there is a 55-gram reduction in infant birth weight or low birth weight for every unit increase of stressful life event [34]. Similar results have been observed elsewhere in European countries [35-37].

In Amsterdam, Paarlberg et al. recruited almost 400 women from several obstetric outpatient clinics to conduct a prospective study on stressors and low birth weight [36]. Questionnaires on daily stressors, psychological and mental well-being, and social support were completed by women throughout their pregnancy. Having experienced daily stressors in the first trimester was associated with an increased risk of low birth weight. Indeed the relationship was strongest when multiple exposures interacted to contribute to a compromised fetal growth. In Scotland expectant mothers perceiving high levels of household stress at 20 weeks gestation had increased odds of low birth weight (OR = 4.7, 95% CI = 1.5 to 13.4) [35]. Results from the Scotland study suggests that the relationship between psychosocial stress and low birth weight may be attributable to variation in energetic intake and expenditure. For example, pregnant women who carry the burden of running a household without the support of a husband or partner may suffer inadequate nutritional provisioning and greater workload, reducing maternal and fetal weight gain.

Overall, preterm birth and low birth weight are commonly studied together as tandem outcomes because infants born preterm are often of low birth weight. It has been estimated that two-thirds of low birth weight infants are born preterm [3]. Prior work in the field had the tendency to combine various psychological processes into one psychosocial category that typically consisted of stress, emotions, coping, social support, and more. However, a growing body of research supports differences in the psychological processes involved in the etiology of both birth outcomes [23,25]. While pregnancy anxiety appears to be a strong predictor of preterm birth, depression and chronic strain appear to be stronger predictors of low birth weight [23]. Epidemiologic and social behavioral studies on the psychological pathways contributing to these two birth outcomes deserve individual attention. Disentangling the components of psychological processes may lead to improved intervention models for at risk populations and better inform health policies that seek to reduce preterm and low birth weight.

Defined as "cognitive and behavioral efforts to manage stressful demands" coping may directly affect birth outcomes, minimize perceived stress, or modify the effects of stress on birth outcomes [23]. However, very little studies exist on the relationship between birth outcomes and coping during pregnancy. A direction for future research may be to consider various coping processes in pregnancy and strategies to effectively reduce anxiety and understand resilience in the face of adversity.

3. Mental health and stress

Stress plays an important role in the development and worsening of mental illness such as depression or anxiety disorders [38-41]. Depression and anxiety are approximately twice as prevalent globally in women as in men [42]. Approximately one in five women will experience depression during her lifetime with the typical age of onset during the reproductive years [43,44]. Estimates on the prevalence of antenatal depression, or depression during pregnancy, can vary depending on the criteria used but can be as high as 16 percent with increasing proportions in the year following delivery [42,45]. The contribution to the Global Burden of Disease (GBD) of only three mental disorders (i.e. mood disorders, schizophrenia and specific anxiety disorders) among women aged 15 to 44 years is seven percent of the total GBD for women of all ages [46]. In fact, depression is fourth among all causes of GBD for women and is expected to rank second by the year 2020.

There has been a growing interest in the potential etiologic association of psychosocial factors, including maternal depression with birth outcomes given a number of studies that support the relationship between stress and maternal depression [47,48]. For example some studies have highlighted the key role of maternal depressive symptoms and general distress during pregnancy on reduced fetal growth, low birth weight and preterm birth [48,49]. The impact of maternal mental disorder on infants goes beyond just delayed psycho-social development but has severe health consequences that are of considerable concern in developing countries. Postpartum non-psychotic depression is the most common complication of childbearing affecting about 10 to 15 percent of all women [50]. The perinatal period is a time of increased physical and emotional demands on expectant or newly mothers and the disability associated with depression can interfere with many essential functions related to both the mothers and infant. Maternal mental health has been associated with reduced breast-feeding, severe malnutrition, stunted growth, increased episodes of diarrhea and lower compliance with immunization schedules [46].

Psychiatric research on pregnancy has largely focused on diagnosable mental disorders such as anxiety and depressive disorders and posttraumatic stress disorder following negative life events or experiences [51]. However, scientific research outside psychiatry has also provided useful information on clinical symptoms during pregnancy using tools such as the Edinburgh Postpartum Depression Scale (EPDS), Beck Depression Inventory, or the Center for Epidemiological Studies Depression Scale [51]. Scores are commonly kept continuous to evaluate symptom severity or often dichotomized to create groups of depressed and non-depressed women as proxy for diagnosed cases. Current understanding of negative affective states during pregnancy and its impact on birth outcomes is mostly based on studies of symptomatology rather than on confirmed diagnoses.

In a recent review, anxiety during pregnancy was identified as a significant predictor of gestational age and preterm birth in seven of 11 studies [23]. Results were more consistent for pregnancy anxiety or pregnancy-specific anxiety which, unlike general state anxiety, is a distinct syndrome reflecting fears about the health and well-being of one's baby, pregnancy, childbirth, and postpartum parenting. One large prospective study of 4,885 births found that women with high pregnancy anxiety had 1.5 times greater risk of a preterm birth after controlling for confounders [22]. Furthermore, pregnancy anxiety predicts risk of spontaneous preterm birth with effect sizes comparable to the effects of known risk factors such as smoking and medical risks [51].

Prior findings on the relationship between antenatal depression and gestational age or preterm birth have been relatively inconsistent and inconclusive [52]. Dunkel Schetter and Glynn reported that 11 out of 14 reviewed studies showed no effect on gestational age due to depressed mood or symptoms of trauma. Furthermore, the three studies that reported association had some methodological limitations [23]. One study from the U.S. had a small sample size of 120 rural women between 16 to 28 weeks gestation and depression symptoms was determined by two screening items [53]. Another study took place in France where 634 pregnant women were assessed using self-administered questionnaires to determine anxiety and depression. Depression was positively associated with spontaneous preterm labor but with large confidence intervals and only among women with a pre-pregnancy body mass index of less than 19 (adjusted OR = 6.9, 95% CI = 1.8 to 26.2) [54]. In a large study, Orr et al. found that women with an elevated depressive symptom score had 1.96 times the odds of experiencing spontaneous preterm birth compared to women with a lower score (95% CI = 1.04 to 3.72) [55]. This U.S. study had a large sample size of 1,399 but only African-American women were included in the study [55].

Due to the conflicting results and limitations related to methodological designs, sample size, biases, and populations studied, Grote et al. conducted a thorough meta-analysis of antenatal depression and the risk of preterm birth, low birth weight, and intrauterine growth restriction [56]. Prospective observational studies in English and non-English languages from 1980 to 2009 were compiled for consideration. A total of 29 articles were included in the analysis. Twenty studies evaluated the association between antenatal depression and preterm birth with relative risk estimates ranging from 1.01 to 4.90. Eleven of the studies showed no significant association but using a random-effects model, depression during pregnancy was significantly associated with preterm birth (RR = 1.13, 96% CI = 1.06-1.21). Furthermore, there was a slightly increased risk for low birth weight (RR=1.18, 95% CI = 1.07-1.30). Thus, antenatal depression, regardless of the type of depression measurement (categorical or continuous) was associated with modest but significant risks of preterm birth and low birth weight. Further, based on categorical measures of antenatal depression, having major depression or clinically significant depressive

http://dx.doi.org/10.5772/54978

symptoms increased the risk of preterm birth by 39%, low birth weight by 49% and intrauterine growth restriction by 45%.

Although the evidence for the association between pregnancy anxiety and gestational age or preterm birth is more robust, depressed mood and chronic strain is often more consistently linked to fetal growth and low birth weight [57]. In a population-based retrospective cohort study of more than 500,000 births in California, psychiatric diagnoses predicted low birth weight after adjusting for marital status, ethnicity, and prenatal care adequacy [58]. In another study of 1,100 women screened for psychiatric disorders during pregnancy, women with a depressive disorder had significantly higher odds of giving birth to infants with low birth weight (OR = 1.82) [59]. Research on the psychological pathways contributing to low gestational age and birth weight deserve individual attention with special emphasis on the type and severity of mood disorders.

Animal models and human studies have also shown that psychosocial and physiological stressors during pregnancy are associated with long term changes in infants' cognitive, physiologic and behavioral outcomes [60-62]. Untreated prenatal depression is the most robust predictor of postpartum depression and has serious consequences for infant and child's development [63]. The most direct evidence comes from animal studies with prenatal exposures to physical stressors such as repeated electrical tail shock, immobilization, noise, and various forms of social stress [64-67]. In other studies using human participants, pregnant women who perceived themselves as stressed gave birth to infants with more difficult behavior, and anxious pregnant women had infants with poor attention regulation in the first year of life [68]. The offspring of women with increased levels of prenatal stress also demonstrated increased restlessness, behavioral problems, and attention regulation issues at two years of age [69]. Untreated postpartum depression leads to chronic recurrent depression and interfere with their children's emotional, behavioral and cognitive well-being later in life [70].

A growing body of evidence indicates that depression during pregnancy is associated with risky behaviors and adverse health practices, such as poor nutrition, delayed prenatal care, adherence to medical recommendations, use of alcohol, cigarettes, and illicit substances which may lead to adverse birth outcomes [58,71-73]. The concomitant effects of depression and stress can influence lifestyle behaviors such as prenatal smoking and cessation behaviors [74]. In fact, one study showed that among pregnant women in the second trimester, smokers were significantly more likely to report depressive symptoms than never-smokers [75]. These lifestyle behaviors could account for a large portion of the risk for adverse birth outcomes. Grote et al. observed smoking had a dose-dependent relationship with preterm birth where smoking more than 10 cigarettes a day increased the likelihood of a early preterm birth of 33-36 weeks by 40 percent and of preterm birth at 32 weeks or less by 60% [56]. In addition, the magnitude of risk for preterm birth and low birth weight posed by antenatal depression was comparable to the risk of smoking 10 or more cigarettes a day. The pharmacological properties of nicotine may serve as a coping strategy for dealing with negative affect among women [76]. Women with psychosocial problems such as depression may be less confident in their changes of successful smoking cessation. Smoking may also provide a quick and direct reinforcement to depressed women with reduced capacities to initiate efforts to quit smoking [77].

4. Mechanisms of stress and preterm birth

There are multiple physiologic pathways that mediate the relationship between prenatal stress and poor birth outcomes. Primary hypothesized mechanisms for the impact of stress on preterm birth are through the neuroendocrine, inflammatory or immune, and behavioral pathways [25].

4.1. Biomedical individualism

Research on chronic stress and pregnancy gathered momentum during the 1990s at which time strong work on psychosocial, neuroendocrine, and preterm birth was generated [1]. Several prospective studies with large sample sizes and standardized measures of stress gave researchers the confidence to proceed with the understanding that stress is a risk factor for preterm delivery although the mechanisms are not fully understood [78]. In contrast, considerably less biopsychosocial research has been conducted on the mechanisms linking stress and low birth weight [3]. Nevertheless, a large proportion of work has focused on two main hypothesized biological mechanisms for preterm birth: the neuroendocrine and inflammatory pathways [78]. Though a smaller subset of preterm birth is attributed to vascular factors, the bulk of existing research has focused on the first two physiological mechanisms [3].

4.2. Physiologic stress response

Experiencing major life events, pregnancy-related anxiety, and racism or discrimination can exacerbate levels of perceived stress among individuals while higher coping skills and greater social support can be protective. While the process may vary depending on the quality (i.e. psychological or physical), strength and duration of stressors, exposure to stress can lead to two physiologic sequence of events involving the autonomic nervous system and hypothalamic-pituitary-adrenal (HPA) axis [1]. Figure 1 depicts the physiologic response to stress as it relates to preterm birth. Corticotrophin-releasing hormone (CRH) plays a key role in initiating and regulating the physiologic stress response. The release of CRH from the hypothalamus to the anterior pituitary initiates the systemic release of adrenocorticotropin hormone (ACTH), which signals the adrenal glands to release glucocorticoids (i.e. cortisol) [1]. Neuronal regulators of the central arousal and systemic sympathetic adrenomedullary systems are innervated to release norepinephrine from a network of neurons throughout the brain resulting in enhanced arousal and increased anxiety [79]. Activation of the autonomic nervous system and HPA axis results in physiologic and behavioral changes characteristic of "fight or flight" responses [80]. The secretion of CRH is down-regulated through a negative feedback loop where increased cortisol levels signal the hypothalamus to reduce further CRH release. Acute or short-term stress prompts the successful return to homeostasis. Long-term activation may indicate the chronic nature of stress or the body's inability to effectively respond to stressors. It has been suggested that constant exposure to stress has cumulative effects of "wear and tear" on the body and this concept of "allostatic load" places individuals at risk for adverse health outcomes such as preterm birth [32,81,82].

http://dx.doi.org/10.5772/54978

4.3. Neuroendocrine

Pregnancy involves significant changes to neuroendocrine, immune, and vascular functioning that affects the uterine environment for fetal development and parturition [83]. In fact, it has been reported that up to 25 percent of preterm births are attributable to the influence of stress on neuroendocrine mechanisms [3]. As described earlier, there are two principal components of the stress response system, the CRH-releasing HPA axis and autonomic nervous system (locus ceruleus-norepinephrine system or LC/NE) [84]. Under stress, the principal regulators of the HPA axis, or CRH and arginine-vasopressin (AVP), are released by the hypothalamus into the hypophyseal portal system leading to the secretion of ACTH by the pituitary. CRH is the most potent agonist for the secretion of ACTH and beta-endorphin from the anterior pituitary. However, in the presence of stress, ACTH can also be regulated by other peptides such as AVP, oxytocin, and vasoactive intestinal peptide [78]. ACTH is transported to the adrenal gland where it stimulates both the synthesis and secretion of glucocorticoids, aldosterone and adrenal androgens [78]. It is interesting to note that there has been growing interest in observed racial and ethnic differences for CRH and ACTH during pregnancy although the mechanisms and reasons for the differences are not well understood [78,85,86].

Circulating levels of CRH-binding protein decrease substantially towards the end of pregnancy resulting in increased levels of plasma CRH [87]. During pregnancy and immediately following birth, maternal hypothalamic CRH secretion is suppressed due to the levels of circulating cortisol; thus, increasing levels of stress-induced CRH may interfere with the hormonal balance [88]. Process variations that underlie fetal growth have an influence on maternal physiologic changes, which in turn, moderate the effect of maternal stress exposure on the developing fetus. This bidirectional relationship between mother and fetus is dynamic and repetitive during pregnancy [89]. Placental CRH plays an important role in preparing for uterine growth and perfusion by communicating between the placenta and adrenal gland to release cortisol into maternal and fetal circulation [78]. In late gestation, cortisol produced by the fetal adrenal cortex blocks the inhibitory effects of progesterone on placental CRH production and leads to a surge in CRH in the placenta [90]. Placental CRH passes directly into the fetus and helps stimulate the fetal adrenal gland directly to increase dehydroepiandrosterone, a precursor for placental estrogen production [91,92]. The conversion to estrogen subsequently affects gap junction formation and oxytocin receptor expression by the myometrium and prostaglandin production that are important events for facilitating uterine contraction and labor [90]. In the presence of chronic or sustained stress, premature or exponential release of CRH gene expression in the placenta may lead to altered physiology of parturition which produces uterine contractions and result in early delivery [93]. This has served as the basis for the placental clock theory under which gene expression and over-production of CRH in the placenta affects gestational length [94]. In addition to prematurity, abnormalities in placental CRH secretion due to stress may be involved in the pathogenesis of fetal growth retardation and preeclampsia – three leading causes of perinatal morbidity and mortality in developed countries [95].

Glucocorticoids exerts a broad range of effects throughout the body, one of which is to inhibit the activation, proliferation, and function of cells involved in immune response [96-98]. Short-term stress prompts the successful return to homeostasis while chronic stimulation of the HPA axis results in hypercortisolemia. Hypercorisolemia is associated with the suppression of growth and sex hormones, a diminished feedback loop, increased risk for a coronary heart disease event, insulin resistance, and obesity [99-102]. In a review of the literature on preterm birth, neuroendocrine markers, and psychosocial factors, Latendresse found that women who had higher plasma concentrations of CRH, ACTH, and cortisol, higher perceived stress or anxiety scores, more risky behaviors like smoking, and lower education were at increased risk for preterm birth [1]. Further, African-American women had higher levels of CRH and were more likely to have preterm infants. In fact, perceived stress and elevated CRH accounted for 20% of the variance in gestational age at birth [103].

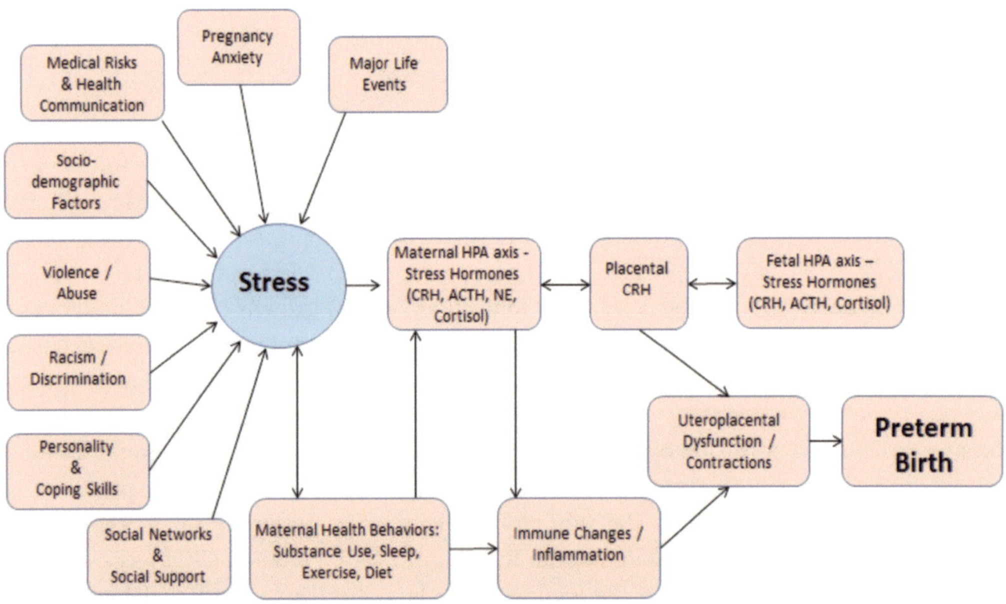

Modified from Dunkel Schetter [3]

Figure 1. Physiologic Stress Response in Relation to Preterm Birth

4.4. Inflammatory/immune system

Maternal and placental hormones also play a role in the inflammatory pathway [87]. It has been reported that repeated episodes of stress can induce a chronic inflammatory process which is associated with inflammatory-related diseases such as atherosclerosis [104]. Inflammation is characterized by an increased production of pro-inflammatory cytokines in response to threats to tissue. The events that regulate homeostasis of the immune system and protective response are coordinated to a large extent by cytokines regulated through type 1 and 2 helper T cells (Th1 and Th2, respectively) [105].

The immune response and inflammation that takes place during the process of fetal implantation is primarily a Th1 response with the secretion of tumor necrosis factor (TNF-β), interferon-gamma (◎-IFN), and interleukins (IL-2) [78]. Since pregnant women only share half of the fetal major histocompatibility complex (MHC) antigens, a certain degree of immunosuppression is required to keep the fetus in the uterus [105]. If the Th1 immune response persisted beyond early implantation, the pregnancy could not be viable. Thus, the immune system cedes to Th2 with a different set of cytokines (i.e. IL-4, IL-10, IL-13) that prevents rejection of fetal implantation by suppressing Th1 and promoting humoral immunity [78]. If this system or balance of cytokines was disrupted, this could lead to an abnormally high production of Th1 pro-inflammatory cytokines (e.g. TNF-α, ◎-IFN) resulting in spontaneous abortion and fetal death. Cytokines produced by Th1 destroys vascular endothelial cells which leaves the embryo vulnerable to ischemic death by increased pro-coagulant secretion [106-108].

Various factors have been known to promote a shift of the pregnancy-protective Th2 cytokine towards a Th1 response resulting in fetal death. For instance, endotoxin is a potent abortogenic substance that stimulates microphages to release cytokines in mice [109]. In addition, the exposure of pregnant mice to a stressor during the implantation period has been known to activate T cells, mast cells, and macrophages in the uterus, resulting in increased secretions of TNF-α [110]. Both pregnancy and stress share a common effect on the immune system – the switch from Th1 to Th2 immunity. Further research is needed to understand the interaction between the two systems to cause disease and elucidate why some people may be more susceptible to adverse birth outcomes or infections.

A psychosocial stress-induced release of glucocorticoids and catecholamines may cause excessive immune response through an exaggerated Th2 response and suppressed Th1 resulting in a greater risk of infection during pregnancy [78]. Reproductive and urinary tract infections, sexually transmitted diseases, and periodontal disease can pose serious risk for preterm birth. For medically indicated causes of preterm birth, stress mediates the promotion of preeclampsia which is also associated with high levels of circulating inflammatory markers [19]. A large proportion of preterm births have been attributed to the inflammatory pathway [111]. Further, high levels of chronic stress have been linked to vaginal bacterial infections at an individual and community level [128]. One must consider the role of genetics in the stress-immune interaction. However, there are no clear or definitive studies that elucidate how the effects of prenatal stress on birth outcomes may be partially mediated by inflammatory processes [3].

5. Fetal programming and life course perspective

Preterm birth is a multifaceted difficult problem and a growing body of work highlights the need for a paradigm shift in considering the interplay of biological, behavioral, psychological, and social factors on improving birth outcomes. The life course perspective may be a useful way to think about maternal stress and preterm birth. This conceptualizes reproductive and birth problems as a result of the culminating experiences and exposures during the life course of the mother [82]. In other words, factors occurring throughout a woman's developmental lifetime, not just during the perinatal period, can alter the quality of the intrauterine environment for her offspring and have a lasting impact on their health. Research in this area has begun to shed light on possible mechanisms through which longitudinal factors produce adverse birth outcomes, such as preterm birth. Two broad mechanisms have been proposed – early programming and cumulative pathway [82].

The early programming model suggests that exposures or experiences (i.e. stressful life events) that occur at a critical period in the developmental process can alter the structure or functioning of an organism or system that becomes manifest in health and risk of disease later in life [82]. Although the biological underpinning for this model is not fully understood, some have attributed this phenomenon to poor fetal nutrition. This notion forms the basis for the Developmental Origins of Adult Disease Hypothesis or Barker's Hypothesis where under-nutrition during gestation increases risk for adult onset diseases [129-131]. Earlier animal models have indicated a critical or sensitive period in early life for the effect of altered fetal nutrition on metabolism, growth, neurodevelopment and major disease [132-136]. Although there are no studies that clearly support programming of reproductive potential, one study came close to relating maternal intrauterine environment to future reproductive outcomes. Lumey et al. found that women exposed in utero to a war-induced famine during the first and second trimesters gave birth to the lowest birth weight infants compared to women who were exposed in utero during the third trimester [137]. Human studies on birth outcomes and cardiovascular disease have also demonstrated that an adverse intrauterine environment can have long-term effects on fetal development and lead to its increased risk for adult-onset chronic disease such as diabetes and hypertension [138,139].

Research indicates a relationship between maternal stress during pregnancy and subsequent cognitive, emotional, and behavioral problems in offspring possibly through the hypothalamic pituitary axes [140-145]. It has been suggested that the association of stress and preterm birth may be mediated by epigenetic changes in the glucocorticoid receptor gene in the developing brain [146]. Perinatal stress is associated with HPA axis hyperreactivity and may be due to feedback resistance as a result of decreased expression of glucocorticoid receptors [147-149]. Mizoguchi et al. observed stress-induced attenuated glucocorticoid negative feedback among animals undergoing chronic stress. Maternal affective disorders have been known to alter fetal HPA axis and physiology [149,150].

As researchers continue to study preterm birth and the role of stress at earlier points in pregnancy or during childhood, this can help elucidate the extent to which maternal stress affects fetal growth and development. For example, in a study by Field et al. on pregnancy anxiety and neonatal behavior, newborns to high anxiety mothers showed more state changes and poor performance on the Brazelton Neonatal Behavior Assessment Scale, which evaluates motor maturity, autonomic stability, and withdrawal [151].

Further, high anxiety mothers had significantly increased prenatal norepinephrine and lower dopamine levels than low anxiety mothers. Further studies have reported that prenatal stress is related to offspring temperament, later behavioral and emotional problems, and worse attention and concentration [68,140,152]. These suggest that maternal stress and affective state can have a significant impact on fetal neuro-development and persist throughout the lifespan of the child [124]. In addition, it shows that fetal brain functioning can be altered by measured maternal neuroendocrine dysregulation which has clinical implications when considering effective interventions to improve health outcomes.

The cumulative pathway model hypothesizes that constant exposure to stress has cumulative effects of "wear and tear" on the body's regulatory process, and this concept of "allostatic load" places individuals at risk for adverse health outcomes such as preterm birth [32,81]. There is still much to be learned on the process of cellular aging and how stress can accelerate the process. However in a landmark study that assessed psychological stress and a proxy for measuring age, Epel et al. found that an accelerated chromosomal telomere shortening was associated with higher levels of perceived stress in premenopausal women caring for their chronically ill children [153]. Telomeres are DNA-protein complexes that cap chromosomal ends and promote stability. Women with the highest level of perceived stress had shorter telomere lengths that were equivalent to aging ten years compared to women with low stress. Further, both perceived stress and long-term exposure to stress was significantly associated with higher oxidative stress and lower telomerase activity. This suggests that chronic stress contributes to increasing allostatic load, resulting in rapid cellular aging and subsequent risk of dysfunction and disease typically associated with older age. The identification of such markers within the context of pregnancy, and in relation to preterm birth could be illuminating.

Chronic and repeated exposure to stress has also been linked to immune-inflammatory dysregulation, insulin resistance, and obesity [99-102]. Suppressed immune system could increase the likelihood of genital tract infections at conception and early pregnancy. Failure to treat pathogens by mid-gestation can lead to preterm labor or premature rupture of membrane [111]. Similarly, overexposure to high levels of glucocorticoids can also lead to exaggerated hyperactive HPA response to stressors which may reflect the inability of the HPA axis to self-regulate [112,113]. Women who experience stress may yield a higher output of norepinephrine and cortisol which could increase CRH gene expression and subsequently lead to preterm birth. These two mechanisms - HPA hyperactivity and immune-inflammatory system – increase the risk for developing cardiovascular diseases, cancers, and experiencing adverse reproductive outcomes.

Several studies relate health disparities in the U.S. to the cumulative differential exposures to damaging physical and social environments [82]. This is evident in studies where preterm birth is a proxy for early health deterioration or "weathering" by age, abuse and trauma, income and poverty [114-116]. For example, Love et al. explored the transgenerational effects of poverty on preterm birth, low birth weight and small for gestational age [116]. Authors found that the age for African-American women to experience the lowest birth weight was less than 20 years which deteriorated with increasing age groups compared to White women whose lowest rate of low birth weight was in their late 20s. The degree of weathering for African

American women, with regards to low birth weight, small for gestational age, and preterm birth, depended on the duration of exposure to low-income neighborhoods and disappeared for those living in non-poor areas. In contrast, no group of white women exhibited weathering even while living in poorer neighborhoods. The biological mechanisms by which a lifetime of differential exposures to discrimination, social inequities and poverty leading to health disparities is not well understood. However, the life course perspective theory frames the issues in such a way that vulnerability to preterm birth or low birth weight is not restricted by time or space, but is all-encompassing, considering the full range of biological, psychological, financial, behavioral and interpersonal stressors and exposures that have become manifested in the widening gap between racial and ethnic groups on many health indicators.

6. Factors that influence stress

There are a multitude of factors that can affect an individual's stress level, including socio-demographic characteristics and environmental and social influences. Stress levels can vary depending on gender, race, life-events, and resiliency. Currently, stress research is fragmented into two mutually exclusive categories – childhood stress and adult or adolescent stress – failing to fully explore the potential connectivity between them. Studies have reported striking evidence on the influence of childhood stressors on neuro-endocrine systems and mental health disorders later in life [117-122]. A recent study by Danese et al. suggested that children exposed to adverse life events, exhibited psychological and physiological abnormalities as adults [123]. This is further documented by DiPietro who reviewed the role of prenatal influences on child neurodevelopment [124]. In addition, Kingston et al. linked childhood stress with prenatal stress which has a significant impact on poor birth outcomes, particularly preterm births [125]. This suggests the significance of a life course pathway to prenatal stress, which in fact includes childhood and adulthood socioeconomic positioning. Furthermore, it alludes to the recent movement in understanding the impact of maternal stress and designing interventions to address the issue of preterm births using the life course perspective [82]. The life course perspective is grounded in the theory that reproductive and poor birth outcomes are the result of the culminating experiences and exposures to stressful assaults during the life course of the mother. The mechanism for this theory is further discussed in the previous section on "Fetal programming and life course perspective".

Although the life course perspective calls for understanding of stress through the life of a prospective mother starting in utero, studies that examine these influences through the developmental stages are lacking. Existing literature predominantly focus on stress during pregnancy and its impact on poor birth outcomes. Various sources have estimated between 25 to 75 percent of women experience stressful life events or social health issues during the antenatal period [20,126]. It has also been reported that about 18 percent of women experience three or more stressful life events during pregnancy [20]. Previous studies have shown that maternal psychosocial stress is associated to education, personality traits, demographic characteristics, and environmental and social influences [2]. Research conducted outside the U.S. reports similar risk factors for stress with regards to age, parity, and prenatal care adequacy [20,127]. Demographic factors such as age, marital discords, intimate partner violence, low education and income are some factors that predispose women to certain levels of stress. Furthermore, stressful life events such as extreme financial distress, death in the family, accidents, injuries, persistent discrimination and other mishaps pose major stress. In fact, most of the psychometric assessments that are validated to measure stress are based on enumerating the occurrence of these life events.

6.1. Lifestyle factors

Stress is known to influence lifestyle behaviors such as smoking, alcohol use, illicit substance use, physical activity and diet. These are also known risk factors for preterm births and relatively amenable to intervention. One of the main preventable causes of preterm births is smoking. Unfortunately, the number of stressful events is inversely associated with smoking cessation. In fact, women reporting three or more stressful events are half as likely to quit smoking compared to women who report no stressful events in the previous year [74]. Smokers during pregnancy tend to be single, of low income, less education and other factors associated with smoking include physical and sexual abuse and high stress levels [154,155]. It has been proposed that since nicotine a vasoconstrictor, reduces the flow of nutrients and oxygen to the developing fetus, this may result in low birth weight infants, reductions in body length and head size, and other perinatal complications [156]. Smokers tend to have less weight gain during pregnancy and in fact, inadequate maternal weight gain has previously been associated with spontaneous preterm delivery and low birth weight infants [157].

High psychosocial stress has also been linked to use of substance, drugs, and alcohol [155,158]. There is considerable evidence on the significant association between acute and chronic stress and substance abuse [159]. It is postulated that people abuse substance and excessively drink alcohol as a means of coping with stressful situations, such as economic stress, marital discourse, and often when there is lack of social support [159-161]. However, the tendency to abuse substances when distressed depends on many factors. Some of the known factors include the intensity and type of stressor, perceived ability to overcome the stressful situation, availability of social support, genetic determinants, and prior history of substance use. Several theories were proposed to understand the role of stress in substance abuse and particularly addiction process. The most frequently cited mechanism was the psychological response to substance abuse that postulates substance abuse or use as a means to cope with stress and in most cases to simply alleviate tension [162-168]. The neurobiological model is another theory that proposes the mechanism for addition. This theory emphasizes the role of incentive sensitization and stress allostasis and provides explanation for craving and loss of control [159,169].

7. Social production of disease/political economy of health

Health disparities among racial and ethnic groups are influenced by the structural, institutional, and interpersonal aspects of society and its health care systems [170]. Stemming from the social analyses of health from the 1830s and emerging in the politically turbulent 1960s and 1970s, this theoretical framework focuses on the "social production of disease" and/or "political economy of health" [171-173]. That is, it addresses economic and political determinants of health and disease and any structural barriers that prevent people from living healthier lives [171-179]. The underlying principle is that economic and political institutions that create, enforce, and perpetuate economic and social privilege and inequality are causes of inequities in health which are also stressors in life [179,180].

Going beyond just healthy choices and behaviors at an individual level, this school of thought takes into consideration significant external forces that perpetuate the disparities in health evident in different populations around the world. For example, disquieting health disparities between Australia's indigenous Aboriginals and the rest of the population has been observed in higher infant mortality rate, more drug abuse and alcoholism, chronic and infectious diseases, and poverty [181]. The average Aboriginal household earns only half of what a typical Australian family earns in a week and poverty has been associated with social problems to varying degrees such as high imprisonment and unemployment rates [182].

Like gender and race, religion forms part of the context that generates stress-inducing social inequities and may influence people's socioeconomic status and health outcomes. Of the 1.6 million Muslims living in the UK, 74% were of Asian ethnic background with smaller proportions of black African Muslims and white British in 2001 [181]. In the US, an estimated 6 to 7 million Muslims is comprised of South Asians (32%), Arabs (26%), and African-Americans (20%) [182]. One study that used aggregate data from 10 different data sources (i.e. World Health Organization, United Nations, UNICEF) indicated significant health disparities between countries with a Muslim majority and non-Muslim majority [184]. National health indicators such as male and female life expectancies, maternal mortality ratio, and infant mortality rate were worse in Muslim majority countries compared to non-Muslim majority countries. Almost half of non-Muslim majority countries were in the high or upper middle income group compared with a quarter of all Muslim majority countries. In fact, annual per capital expenditure on health in Muslim majority countries was a fifth of that in non-Muslim majority countries. Additionally, gross national income, literacy rate, access to clean water, and government corruption accounted for 52 to 72 percent of the differences in health outcomes between the two groups. The gradient in health within and between countries can be linked to the unequal distribution of power, income and goods or services. The structural determinants and conditions of daily life make up the social determinants of health, and can account for a large portion of the health inequities observed within and between countries [184].

Discrimination and poverty pose serious challenges in closing the health gaps between racial and ethnic groups. Following the fall of Apartheid South African's Government of National Unity defined and proposed five key developmental priorities to work towards rebuilding the community: employment, housing, education, nutrition, and health [185]. Nearly two decades later, racial and economic discrimination undermine the progress and development in achieving these goals. Racial group still appear to be a strong determinant of income, education, health care coverage, and the quality of medical treatment [186,187]. Similarly, using data from a national survey, Charasse et al. reported that even after controlling for important socio-demographic characteristics, Whites and Africans did not share the same level of health risks [185]. Authors found that Whites tended to have higher income, better education, and more favorable health status than Africans.

A large population-based survey of newly mothers in Australia also highlight a concerning level of social adversity associated with stressful life events and social health problems during pregnancy [20]. One in six women reported experienced three or more stressful life events or social health issues in the 12 months preceding the birth. Women who experienced more life events and social health problems were significantly more likely to report discrimination in the health care settings (OR = 2.69, 95% CI = 2.2 to 3.3) and had a twofold increased odds of having a low birth weight infant compared with women reporting no social health issues. They were also more likely to have antenatal care later in pregnancy and with fewer visits.

Over the past 50 years, improved and expanded prenatal care has resulted in the identification of high-risk pregnancies, leading to an overall reduction of infant mortality in the United States. In the early 1900s, 100 infants died for every 1,000 live births before reaching their first birthday [188]. Since then, the infant mortality rate has declined by more than 90 percent to a rate of 7.2 deaths per 1,000 live births in 2000 [189]. However, African-Americans have been disproportionately affected by the problem. Preliminary results from the U.S. Centers for Disease Control and Prevention showed that the mortality rate for black infants was 11.6 deaths per 1,000 live births compared with 5.2 deaths per 1,000 live births among white infants [190]. In short, black infants die at 2.2 times the rate of white infants within the first year of life. Even after controlling for socio-demographic factors, African Americans with adequate prenatal care still have poorer birth outcomes than their White counterparts [188].

In the U.S., African American women are more likely to die from pregnancy-related complications, have preterm or low birth weight infants, deliver an infant with congenital anomalies, experience a spontaneous abortion and ectopic pregnancy compared to women of other racial and ethnic backgrounds [191-196]. The influence of income on adverse pregnancy outcomes has been previously examined in military populations where pregnant women do not necessarily have financial barriers to health care. Although black women in the military have better pregnancy outcomes than black women in the general population, disparities persist between black and white enlisted women [197]. Furthermore, disparate birth outcomes are evident even among those who are college-educated. Although education is known to be a protective factor against adverse birth outcomes, black women with higher education experience disproportionately high rates of low birth weight compared to college-educated white women [198]. These disparities underscore the need to consider factors other than socioeconomic status to account for the health disparities.

Speculations that racial disparities in adverse health outcomes is attributable to genetic factors have been contradicted by studies that found black immigrants from African or Caribbean do not experience the same rates of adverse pregnancy outcomes as African-Americans from the U.S., in fact, they begin to show worse health outcomes the longer they live in the U.S. [199-201] Racial disparities in adverse outcomes has spurred interest in the role of psychosocial factors such as stress in pregnancy [202]. It has been previously documented that African American women report a greater number of life events and are more distressed by them than any other racial or ethnic groups [25,203]. Racism can be conceptualized as an individual-level psychosocial stressor and is defined as a multidimensional construct that involves the oppression and denigration of individuals by other individuals and social institutions on the basis of skin color or membership in a particular ethnic group [204].

Perceived racism across the lifetime is a significant predictor of birth weight in African Americans and may account for racial differences in infant mortality rates [205]. Preterm birth is also suggested to occur in the context of social and economic structures such as acculturation stress, racism, and poverty [2]. For example, a small prospective observational study was conducted to examine the roles that general, pregnancy, and racism stress play in racial differences in birth outcomes (birth weight and gestational age) [205]. Perceived racism and indicators of general stress were associated with low birth weight. Lifetime and childhood indicators of perceived racism predicted birth weight and attenuated racial differences independent of medical and socio-demographic variables.

The stress of perceived racism and discrimination, differences in how the health care system responds to individuals of different racial backgrounds should be further evaluated to address the slow progress in closing the large health gap between racial and ethnic groups. While it is important to acknowledge the role of individual factors such as discrimination and racism on prematurity and low birth weight, this problem is multifaceted and should compel policy-makers, social services, and health care providers to recognize all the other behavioral, medical, social, environmental, and institutional factors that contribute to the persistent racial and ethnic health disparities. Efforts to reduce discrimination and racism must be taken in the context of ensuring safe neighborhoods, access to healthy food, quality and culturally sensitive medical care to have high impact on such a complex problem. Intervention efforts to improve birth outcomes in the U.S. have had limited success, in part, due to a focus on individual level programs that fail to consider contexts affecting maternal and child health, including neighborhood exposures [206-208]. This necessitates support for social and health programs that provide more comprehensive care for women. Recognizing this need, programs have been designed and implemented to address some of the social determinants. For instance, The Healthy Start program is a U.S. federally-funded initiative to reduce the national infant mortality rate and improve perinatal outcomes by leveraging community resources and workers [209].

8. Measurements

In order to fully understand the role of stress on perinatal health, it is important to effectively quantify and measure its characteristics. Defining or measuring stress can be confusing due to the differences in nature and duration of exposure. Identifying the impact on high-risk populations and the correct manner in which to assess stress poses a great task for researchers. Prior research highlights the importance of differentiating between global stress and pregnancy-specific stress in order to better understand and identify the impact of prenatal stress on maternal and infant health outcomes [210]. Pregnancy-specific stress is defined as the emotional response to the stressfulness of pregnancy itself [210]. It has been suggested that pregnancy-specific stress may have a more deleterious impact on birth outcomes such as preterm birth [210]. Differences between the types of stress and how they contribute to poor birth outcomes has yet to be fully explored.

Previous work yield many different stress measures, however, the most commonly used instruments can be classified into four domains based on a construct published elsewhere – external, perceived, enhancers, and buffers [21]. Examples of external stressors include life events or daily hassles; perceived stress reflect perceptions of racial or gender discrimination and other subjective stress levels; enhancers of stress include anxiety or depression; and buffers of stress cover social support systems and coping mechanisms [4,21]. General stressful life events measures (e.g. General Health Questionnaire and Perceived Stress Scale and pregnancy-specific stress instruments (e.g. Pregnancy Experience Scale, Pregnancy-Related Anxiety Questionnaire, Pregnancy-Related Anxiety Scale, Pregnancy-Specific Anxiety Scale, Prenatal Distress Questionnaire, and Prenatal Social Environment Inventory) have been used throughout literature [210,211,219]. Table 1 summarizes commonly used measures for experiencing global or pregnancy-specific stress.

8.1. General Health Questionnaire (GHQ)

Originally developed by Goldberg the General Health Questionnaire (GHQ) is a widely used instrument for measuring general psychological health in community settings and non-psychiatric clinical settings such as primary care [211]. In general the GHQ focuses on two main classes of phenomena: inability to carry out one's normal healthy functions; and emergence of new phenomena that are distressing [212]. Translated into 38 different languages and available in a variety of versions using 12, 28, 30, or 60 items, this instrument demonstrates high reliability and validity in many different populations with reliability and correlation coefficients ranging from 0.78 to 0.95 [213-216] and 0.35 to 0.79 [217-218], respectively. The 12- items GHQ is one of the most extensively used screening instrument for common mental disorders [219] and its brevity makes it an attractive choice for use in busy clinical settings and for patients who need help to complete the questionnaire [220]. Responses to each item ranges from zero (not at all) to three (much more than usual) with a total possible score based on the version allowing for means and distributions to be calculated.

8.2. Perceived stress scale

The Perceived Stress Scale (PSS) is one of the most widely-used psychological instruments for measuring the perception of stress [221]. The scale includes a number of questions about the level of experienced stress over the previous month and has three versions with 14, 10, and four items, respectively. The PSS prompts subjects to rate on a scale from zero (never) to four (very often) how often they have perceived an event or negative feeling in the past month. This tool demonstrates strong internal consistency, with a Cronbach's alpha ranging from 0.75 to

0.91 [221-223]. It also has the virtues of being brief, easy to understand, and assessing stress response in the general population on a continuum from relatively mild to severe forms of stress.

Similar to other non-specific stress measures, a major limitation of GHQ and PSS is the failure to differentiate between general stress and pregnancy-specific stress. Although pregnancy-specific stress may occur concomitantly to general or non-specific stress, research suggests that pregnancy-specific stress may be particularly more potent and have serious implications on birth outcomes [34,61,68,224,225]. For example, Roesch et al. found that pregnancy anxiety predicted earlier birth while general state anxiety and general perceived stress did not [225]. The timing of prenatal stress exposure may also be of importance. In one study, researchers found that stress experienced during the second trimester was more predictive of preterm delivery than exposure to stress later in the pregnancy [27]. Several studies have shown a decline in psychological and physiological stress response in pregnant women as pregnancy progresses [28-30]. For example, Glynn et al. reported that pregnant women who experienced the 1994 Northridge earthquake in California showed a differential emotional response to the earthquake depending on their gestational age at the time of the event [28]. There was a significant association between women who experienced the stress early in the pregnancy and shorter gestational age at delivery. Participants in the first trimester also evaluated the earthquake as more upsetting and aversive than women in the second or third trimester scoring higher on a life events inventory. Considering the type of stress and time frame of maternal exposure to stress may be useful in understanding the impact on developing fetus.

Measure	Description	Number of Items	Scale Type	*Cronbach's Alpha	€Test-retest Reliability
General Health Questionnaire	Screening tool for detecting non-specific psychiatric illness through items that address the inability to perform daily activities and feelings of distress	12, 28, 30, 60	4-point	0.78 - 0.95	0.35 - 0.79
Perceived Stress Scale	Measures the degree to which situations in one's life over the past month are appraised as stressful (i.e. unpredictable, uncontrollable, and overloading)	4, 10, 14	5-point	0.75 - 0.91	0.85 (over two days)
Pregnancy Experience Scale (hassles subscale)	A measure containing two subscales of which the "hassles" subscale is intended to reflect the daily challenges related to pregnancy (frequency and intensity of hassles)	20	4-point	0.91 - 0.95	frequency 0.57 - 0.83; intensity 0.61 - 0.76

Measure	Description	Number of Items	Scale Type	*Cronbach's Alpha	€Test-retest Reliability
Pregnancy-Related Anxiety Questionnaire-Revised	Measures specific fears and worries related to pregnancy (i.e. delivery, infant health, and egocentric feelings/fear of change)	34	5-point	0.73 - 0.88	0.56 - 0.76
Pregnancy-Related Anxiety Scale	Items assess the extent to which participants worry or feel concerned about their health, baby's health, labor and delivery, and postpartum infant care	10	4-point	0.70 - 0.85	0.83
Pregnancy-Specific Anxiety Scale	Includes pregnancy-specific anxiety items that addresses maternal affective states during pregnancy	4	5-point	0.51 – 0.72	0.56 - 0.68
Prenatal Distress Questionnaire	Evaluates the most common concerns of pregnant women relating to birth and baby, weight and body image, and emotions and relationships	12	5-point	0.80 - 0.81	0.75
Prenatal Social Environment Inventory	Items cover potential stressors over the past 12 months associated with family and marital relationships, health, pregnancy, work, neighborhood, parenting, and finances	41	Yes/No	0.80	0.73

* Cronbach's alpha (internal consistency reliability) is a measure of inter-item correlations

€ Test-retest reliability (correlation coefficient) is a measure of stability over time

Table 1. Commonly used general and pregnancy-specific stress measures

8.3. Pregnancy Experience Scale (PES)

The PES [226] was developed in 1999 to evaluate maternal appraisal of positive and negative stressors during pregnancy, with reliability and validity data reported within later studies [61,224,227]. The scale aimed to reflect the daily minor challenges and positive emotions experienced by pregnant women. The scale consists of 41 items of which 20 are in the hassles subscale. Questions on discomforts of pregnancy, body changes, relationships, and concerns about the infant are among the topics specific to pregnancy-related stress. Respondents are directed to indicate whether each item is a hassle and/or an uplift on a four-point Likert scale, ranging from zero (not at all) to three (a great deal). In addition to calculating the frequency and intensity of hassles and uplifts scores, a composite ratio score of positive to negative experiences in pregnancy can be ascertained with values greater than one indicating more hassles and scores lower than one indicating more uplifts than hassles. The alpha internal reliability rating ranges between 0.91 and 0.95 [212]. Authors wanted to challenge research that focused too narrowly on just the distressing aspects of pregnancy by also considering the role of positive emotions in fostering good pregnancy outcomes.

8.4. Pregnancy-Related Anxiety Questionnaire-Revised (PRAQ-R)

The Pregnancy-Related Anxiety Questionnaire was a 55 item measure developed by Van den Bergh in 1990 that addressed common pregnancy fears (e.g. fear for delivery and baby's health) which led to a shorter version (PRAQ-R) that later became available in 2002 [68,228]. PRAQ-R consists of 34 items with responses to questions on a five point scale ranging from "never" to "very often". PRAQ-R presents good internal consistency and convergent validity data with general stress or anxiety measures. Further analysis of PRAQ-R shows a test-retest reliability rating of 0.56-0.76 and a range in alpha internal reliability rating of 0.73-0.88 [68,152]. No predictive validity data related to preterm birth has been reported to date. Given that PRAQ and PRAQ-R were designed using low-risk populations in Belgium and Netherlands, the applicability to other more diverse communities may be limited.

8.5. Pregnancy-Related Anxiety Scale (PRAS)

Rini et al. revised the PRAS with the goal of linking psychological stress and birth outcome [34,229]. The revised PRAS was used to assess the association between prenatal psychosocial stress, personal resources, sociocultural context, and infant birth weight and gestational age at birth. This was done by having respondents complete a ten item scale assessing their level of stress surrounding various pregnancy related situations; responses were on a four-point Likert scale, ranging from never or not at all, to a lot of the time or very much. There is no recall period for the PRAS because it asks how the respondent is feeling at present time. The internal reliability of the revised version of PRAS in English and Spanish ranged from 0.70 to 0.85 [210, 229]. One aspect of the PRAS that is seldom seen in stress measures is the stress surrounding the mother's thoughts regarding her pregnancy. Stress generated by a mother's thoughts about the pregnancy and birth is an important component in maternal stress research.

8.6. Pregnancy-Specific Anxiety Scale (PSAS)

Developed at the University of California, Los Angeles, the Pregnancy-Specific Anxiety Scale (PSAS) is composed of four pregnancy-specific anxiety items derived from a factor analysis of a larger pool of items that addressed maternal affective states during pregnancy [225]. In the first study that reported using PSAS to find associations with gestational age, participants were encouraged to talk about how they felt about being pregnant and asked to indicate how often they felt anxious, concerned, afraid or panicky in the previous week. All responses were provided on a 5-point scale ranging from one (not at all) to five (very much). It was determined that pregnancy-specific anxiety was associated with shorter gestation age after controlling for known risk factors. Further analysis of PSAS in Canada and in the U.S. shows a test-retest reliability rating of 0.56-0.68 and a range in alpha internal reliability rating of 0.51-0.72 [225,230-232]. Poor internal consistency, lack of correlation to physiological measures of stress, and failure to replicate findings in African-American populations are noteworthy limitations.

8.7. Prenatal Distress Questionnaire (PDQ)

Originally reported by Yali and Lobel in 1999, the 12-item Prenatal Distress Questionnaire (PDQ) was created and tested in a pilot to create pregnancy-specific distress scores [126]. Participants were asked to indicate how concerned or worried they were about their pregnancy on a five-point scale ranging from zero (not at all) to four (extremely). Questions pertained to three main types of concerns: birth and baby, weight and body image, and emotions and relationships [235]. Responses were then summed to create a total pregnancy-specific distress score for each individual. Several studies from the US, Germany and UK have provided reliability and validity data on the instrument. With an alpha internal reliability rating range of 0.80 - 0.81 and a test-retest reliability rating of 0.75, the PDQ demonstrates good internal consistency [127,234-236].

8.8. Prenatal Social Environment Inventory (PSEI)

In 1992, Suezanne Orr and her colleagues developed the PSEI to address limitations from the use of other life events inventories [237]. Such drawbacks were the inclusion of items that would prove to be inapplicable to certain subgroups, as well as assessing chronic stressors with the use of lengthy instruments, or instruments that are not germane to some subgroups. The PSEI consists of 41, yes or no questions, assessing stress in the past year. The 30-day test-retest reliability rating was 0.73 and the alpha internal reliability rating was 0.80. While the PSEI samples a wide variety of potential stressors, the range of information obtained with its yes or no response, is limited. In essence, the PSEI is a good measure of the prevalence of potentially stressful events in the past year, but lacks the ability to obtain qualitative data on the effects of those stressful events on the respondent.

Although some pregnancy-specific stress measures are able to predict adverse outcomes, the theoretical underpinnings of measures are lacking and largely undocumented in the literature [210]. Further consideration of theoretical models in stress measurement development can help build confidence in the use of pregnancy-specific stress measures for studies and lead to more effective stress reduction interventions that target specific concerns and groups of women rather than global and untailored interventions. Furthermore, inconsistent use of measures and definitions to assess stress has been a challenge in accurately understanding its health consequences. While interviews are useful for minimizing missing data by connecting with study participants, stress is often assessed by asking an individual to recall events that have occurred in either the distant or recent past. This introduces recall bias and compromises the reliability of the measure. Questionnaires and interviews are also subjective means to ascertain stress that may be prone to recall bias. However, the possibility of bias should not be grounds for rejection of a stress measure, rather, it should be considered in any conclusions drawn from the data.

Scientific advancements have uncovered possible biological markers (or biomarkers) of stress that provide objective and quantifiable measures, and solutions to the difficulties of qualitatively measuring stress. Biomarkers are defined by Hulk et al. as "cellular, biochemical or molecular alterations…in biological media such as human tissues, cells, or fluids" [238]. These biomarkers that are obtained from saliva, urine, and plasma may provide an objective measure for understanding the cause, progression, and worsening of maternal stress [239]. For example, maternal levels of cortisol, C-reactive protein, and alpha-amylase have been identified as markers for stress and possible biological mechanisms associated with the increased risk for pregnancy complications and preterm birth [240-242]. These markers include the use of technologies that expand people's understanding on the underlying pathogenesis of preterm birth and risk factors [243]. In epidemiologic or medical research, biomarkers address the need for more direct measurement of exposures in the causal pathway of disease that is free from recall bias and improved validity [244].

9. Conclusion

Stress is an important risk factor affecting preterm birth. Despite the growing literature, there are gaps that need to be addressed. Definitive studies that link stress, inflammation, and preterm birth need to be further explored. Specifically, more research is needed to assess pregnancy anxiety and its mediating effects on early birth. Indeed, stress pathways may be an entry point to other vascular and inflammatory pathways leading to premature delivery and low birth weight [78]. Many studies report the deleterious effects of stress on the fetal neurodevelopmental process that may have repercussions even into childhood. Arguments for the life course perspective or social productions of disease are alternative explanations that move the discussion beyond just individual choices and behaviors. The problem is complex and requires a multifaceted approach to come to meaningful and realistic solutions. In addition, there is a need for more research in coping, resiliency and other stress management techniques during pregnancy [3]. While studies that explore the effects of stress on birth outcomes are important, more is needed to develop and test interventions or prevention programs with respect to a positive impact on birth outcomes [1]. Health care providers can be better informed to refer patients to appropriate resources and supplemental services. Social support interventions need to be guided by predictive models and more needs to be done to elucidate which components of interventions account for the largest variability in birth outcomes. Lastly, more work can be done to evaluate how physiologic responses to stressors might account for health disparities [245]. Progress in improving birth outcomes is undermined by growing health disparities between various sub-populations. This should compel policymakers and health care providers to recognize all the other behavioral, medical, social, environmental, and institutional factors that contribute to persistent racial and ethnic health disparities.

Author details

Susan Cha[1] and Saba W. Masho[1,2]

1 Department of Epidemiology and Community Health, School of Medicine, Virginia Commonwealth University, USA

2 Department of Obstetrics and Gynecology, School of Medicine, Virginia Commonwealth University, USA

References

[1] Latendresse, G. The interaction between chronic stress and pregnancy: Preterm birth from a biobehavioral perspective. J Midwifery Wom Heal. (2009). , 54, 8-17.

[2] Cohen, S, Kessler, R, & Gordon, L. Measuring Stress: A Guide for Health and Social Scientists (1st ed.). New York: Oxford University Press; (1997).

[3] Dunkel Schetter CPsychological science on pregnancy: Stress processes, biopsychosocial models, and emerging research issues. Annu Rev Psychol. (2011).

[4] Chen, M. J, Grobman, W. A, & Gollan, J. K. Borders AEB. The use of psychosocial stress scales in preterm birth research. AJOG. (2011). , 205, 402-434.

[5] Wilson-costello, D, Friedman, H, Minich, N, Fanaroff, A. A, & Hack, M. Improved survival rates with increased neurodevelopmental disability for extremely low birth weight infants in the 1990s. Pediatrics. (2005). , 115(4), 997-1003.

[6] Allen, M. C, & Jones, M. D. Medical complications of prematurity. Obstet Gynecol. (1986). , 67(3), 427-437.

[7] Christian, L. M. Psychoneuroimmunology in pregnancy: Immune pathways linking stress with maternal health, adverse birth outcomes, and fetal development. Neurosci Biobehav R. (2012).

[8] Carmichael, S. L, & Shaw, G. M. Maternal life event stress and congenital anomalies. Epidemiology. (2000). , 11, 30-35.

[9] Hare, O, & Creed, T. F. Life events and miscarriage. British Journal of psychiatry. (1995).

[10] Wisborg, K, Barklin, A, Hedegaard, M, & Henriksen, T. B. Psychological stress during pregnancy and stillbirth: Prospective study. BJOG-Int J Obstet Gy. (2008).

[11] Abeysena, C, Jayawardana, P, & Seneviratne, R. Effect of psychosocial stress on maternal complications during pregnancy: A cohort study. International Journal of Collaborative Research on Internal Medicine Public Health. (2010).

[12] Goldenberg, R. L, Culhane, J. F, Iams, J. D, & Romero, R. Epidemiology and causes of preterm birth. Lancet. (2008). , 371, 75-84.

[13] Mathews, T. J, & Menacker, F. MacDorman MF. Infant mortality statistics from the 2002 period. Mon Vital Stat Rep. (2004). , 53, 1-29.

[14] Martin, J. A, Hamilton, B. E, Sutton, P. D, Ventura, S. J, Menacker, F, & Munson, M. L. Births: Final data for 2003. National Vital Statistics Reports. (2005). , 54(2), 1-116.

[15] Lobel, M, Cannella, D. L, Graham, J. E, Devincent, C, Schneider, J, & Meyer, B. A. Pregnancy-specific stress, prenatal health behaviors, and birth outcomes. Health Psychol. (2008).

[16] Sontag, L. W. Significance of fetal environmental differences. Am J Obstet Gynecol. (1941). , 42, 996-1003.

[17] Gunter, L. M. Psychopathology and stress in the life experience of mothers of premature infants. A Comparative study. Am J Obstet Gynecol. (1963). , 86, 333-340.

[18] Lobel, M. Dunkel Schetter C. Conceptualizing stress to study effects on health: Environmental, perceptual, and emotional components. Anxiety Research. (1990). , 3, 213-230.

[19] Hedegaard, M, Henriksen, T. B, Sabroe, S, & Secher, N. J. Psychological distress in pregnancy and preterm delivery. Brit Med J. (1993). , 307, 234-239.

[20] Brown, S. J, Yelland, J. S, Sutherland, G. A, Baghurst, P. A, & Robinson, J. S. Stressful life events, social health issues and low birthweight in an Australian population-based birth cohort: Challenges and opportunities in antenatal care. BMC Public Health. (2011).

[21] Dole, N, Savitz, D. A, & Hertz-picciotto, I. Siega-Riz Am, McMahon MJ, Buekens P. Maternal stress and preterm birth. Am J Epidemiol. (2003). , 157, 14-24.

[22] Kramer, M. S, Lydon, J, Seguin, L, et al. Stress pathways to spontaneous preterm birth: The role of stressors, psychological distress, and stress hormones. Am J Epidemiol. (2009).

[23] Dunkel Schetter CGlynn L. Stress in pregnancy: empirical evidence and theoretical issues to guide interdisciplinary researchers. In: Contrada R, Baum A, eds. Handbook of stress science: biology, psychology, and health. New York, NY: Springer Publishing Company; (2011). , 321-343.

[24] Lobel, M. Dunkel Schetter C, Scrimshaw SC. Prenatal maternal stress and prematurity: A prospective study of socioeconomically disadvantaged women. Health Psychol. (1992). , 11, 32-40.

[25] Zambrana, R. E. Dunkel Schetter C, Collins C, Scrimshaw SC. Mediators of ethnic-associated differences in infant birth weight. J Urban health. (1999). , 76, 102-116.

[26] Hobel, C. J, Goldstein, A, & Barrett, E. S. Psychosocial stress and pregnancy outcome. Clin Obstet Gynecol. (2008).

[27] Class, Q. A, Lichtenstein, P, Langstrom, N, & Onofrio, D. BM. Timing of prenatal maternal exposure to severe life events and adverse pregnancy outcomes: A population study of 2.6 million pregnancies. Psychosom Med. (2011). , 73(3), 234-241.

[28] Glynn, L. M, & Wadhwa, P. D. Dunkel Schetter C, et al. When stress happens matters: Effects of earthquake timing on stress responsivity in pregnancy. Am J Obstet Gynecol. (2001). , 184, 637-642.

[29] DiPietro JACostigan KA, Gurewitsch ED. Maternal psychophysiological change during the second half of gestation. Biol Psychol. (2005). , 69, 23-38.

[30] Kammerer, M, Adams, D, Von Castelberg, B, & Glover, V. Pregnant women become insensitive to cold stress. BMC Pregnancy Childbirth. (2002).

[31] Lederman, S. A, Rauh, V, Weiss, L, et al. The effects of the World Trade Center event on birth outcomes among term deliveries at three lower Manhattan hospitals. Environ Health Perspect. (2004). , 112, 1772-1778.

[32] Rich-edwards, J. W, & Grizzard, T. A. Psychosocial stress and neuroendocrine mechanisms of preterm delivery. Am J Obstet Gynecol. (2005). S, 30-35.

[33] Borders AEBGrobman WA, Amsden LB, Holl JL. Chronic stress and low birth weight neonates in a low-income population of women. Obstet Gynecol. (2007). , 109, 331-38.

[34] Wadhwa, P. D, Sandman, C. A, & Porto, M. Dunkel Schetter C, Garite TJ. The association between prenatal stress and infant birth weight and gestational age at birth: A prospective investigation. Am J Obstet Gynecol. (1993). , 169, 858-865.

[35] Pritchard, C. W, & Teo, P. Y. Preterm birth, low birthweight and the stressfulness of the household role for pregnant womcn. Soc Sci Med. (1994). , 38, 89-96.

[36] Paarlberg, K. M, Vingerhoets, A. J, Passchier, J, Dekker, G. A, Heinen, A. G, & Van Geijn, H. P. Psychosocial predictors of low birth weight: A prospective study. Br J Obstet Gynaecol. (1999). , 106, 834-841.

[37] Grjibovski, A, Bygren, L. O, Svartbo, B, et al. Housing conditions, perceived stress, smoking, and alcohol: Determinants of fetal growth in Northwest Russia. Acta Obstet Gynecol Scand. (2004). , 83, 1159-1166.

[38] Kessler, R. C. The effects of stressful life events on depression. Annu Rev Psychol. (1997). , 48, 191-214.

[39] Kendler, K. S, Hettema, J. M, Butera, F, Gardner, C. O, & Prescott, C. A. Life events dimensions of loss, humiliation, entrapment, and danger in the prediction of onsets of major depression and generalized anxiety. Arch Gen Psychiatry. (2003). , 60, 789-796.

[40] Uliaszek, A. A, Zinbarg, R. E, Mineka, S, et al. A longitudinal examination of stress generation in depressive and anxiety disorders. J Abnorm Psychol. (2012). , 121(1), 4-1.

[41] Yoon, K. L, & Joormann, J. Stress reactivity in social anxiety disorder with and without comorbid depression. J Abnorm Psychol. (2012). , 121(1), 250-255.

[42] World Health OrganizationMental Health. Available at: http://www.who.int/mental_health/prevention/suicide/MaternalMH/en/index.html.Accessed July 31, (2012).

[43] Weissman, M. M. Advances in psychiatric epidemiology: Rates and risks for major depression. Am J Public Health. (1987). , 77, 445-451.

[44] Weissman, M. M, & Olfson, M. Depression in women: Implications for health care research. Science. (1995). , 269, 799-801.

[45] Leight, K. L, Fitelson, E. M, Weston, C. A, & Wisner, K. L. Childbirth and mental disorders. Int Rev Psychiatr. (2010). , 22, 453-471.

[46] World Health OrganizationMaternal mental health and child health and development in low and middle income countries. http://www.who.int/mental_health/prevention/suicide/mmh_jan08_meeting_report.pdf.Published (2008). Accessed July 31, 2012.

[47] Kendler, K. S, Karkowski, L. M, & Prescott, C. A. Causal relationship between stressful life events and the onset of major depression. Am J Psychiatry. (1999).

[48] Dayan, J, Creveuil, C, Marks, M. N, et al. Prenatal depression, prenatal anxiety, and spontaneous preterm birth: a prospective cohort study among women with early and regular care. Psychosom Med. (2006).

[49] Field, T, Diego, M, & Hernandez-reif, M. Prenatal depression effects on the fetus and newborn: A review. Infant Behav Dev. (2006). , 29, 445-455.

[50] Warner, R, Appleby, L, Whitton, A, & Faragher, B. Demographic and obstetric risk factors for postnatal psychiatric morbidity. British Journal of Psychiatry. (1996). , 168, 607-611.

[51] Dunkel Schetter CTanner L. Anxiety, depression and stress in pregnancy: Implications for mothers, children, research, and practice. Curr Opin Psychiatr. (2012). , 25(2), 141-148.

[52] Yonkers, K, Wisner, K, Stewart, D, et al. Management of depression during pregnancy: A report from the American Psychiatric Association and the American College of Obstetricians and Gynecologists. Gen Hosp Psychiatry. (2009). , 31(5), 403-413.

[53] Jesse, E, Seaver, W, & Wallace, D. Maternal psychosocial risks predict preterm birth in a group of women from Appalachia. Midwifery. (2003). , 19, 191-202.

[54] Dayan, J, Creveuil, C, Herlicoviez, M, et al. Role of anxiety and depression in the onset of spontaneous preterm labor. Am J Epidemiol. (2002). , 155(4), 293-301.

[55] Orr, S, & James, S. Blackmore Prince C. Maternal prenatal depressive symptoms and spontaneous preterm birth among African-American women in Baltimore, Maryland. Am J Epidemiol. (2002). , 156(9), 797-802.

[56] Grote, N. K, Bridge, J. A, Gaven, A. R, Melville, J. L, Iyengar, S, & Katon, W. J. A meta-analysis of depression during pregnancy and the risk of preterm birth, low birth weight, and intrauterine growth restriction. Arch Gen Psychiatry. (2010). , 67(10), 1012-1024.

[57] Diego, M, Jones, N, Field, T, et al. Maternal psychological distress, prenatal cortisol, and fetal weight. Psychosom Med. (2006). , 68, 747-753.

[58] Kelly, R. H, Russo, J, Holt, V. L, et al. Psychiatric and substance use disorders as risk factors for low birth weight and preterm delivery. Obstet Gynecol. (2002). , 100(2), 297-304.

[59] Rogal, S, Poschman, K, Belanger, K, et al. Effects of posttraumatic stress disorder on pregnancy outcomes. J Affect Disord. (2007). , 102, 137-43.

[60] Connor, O, & Heron, T. G. J, Vivette Glover. Antenatal anxiety predicts child behavioral/emotional problems independently of postnatal depression. J Am Acad Child Psy. (2002). , 41(12), 1470-1477.

[61] DiPietro JAGhera MM, Costigan K, Hawkins M. Measuring the ups and downs of pregnancy stress. J Psychosom Obstet Gynaecol. (2004). , 25, 189-201.

[62] Sjostrom, K, Valentin, L, Thelin, T, & Marsal, K. Maternal anxiety in late pregnancy: Effect on fetal movements and fetal heart rate. Early Hum Dev. (2002). , 67, 87-100.

[63] Robertson, E, Celasun, N, & Stewart, D. E. (2003). Risk factors for postpartum depression. In Stewart, D.E., Robertson, E., Dennis, C.-L., Grace, S.L., & Wallington, T. (2003). Postpartum depression: Literature review of risk factors and interventions.

[64] Takahashi, L. K, Baker, E. W, & Kalin, N. H. Ontogeny of behavioral and hormonal responses to stress in prenatally stressed male rat pups. Physiol Behav. (1990). , 47, 357-364.

[65] Ward, I. L, & Weisz, J. Differential effects of maternal stress on circulating levels of corticosterone, progesterone and testosterone in male and female rat fetuses and their mothers. Endocrinology. (1984). , 114, 1635-1644.

[66] Clarke, A. S, & Schneider, M. L. Prenatal stress has long-term effects on behavioral response to stress in juvenile rhesus monkeys. Dev Psychobiol. (1993). , 26, 293-304.

[67] Schneider, M. L, & Coe, C. L. Repeated social stress during pregnancy impairs neuromotor development of the primate infant. J Devel Behav Pediatr. (1993). , 14, 81-87.

[68] Huizink, A. C, De Medina, P. G, Mulder, E. J, Visser, G. H, & Buitelaar, J. K. Psychological measures of prenatal stress as predictors of infant temperament. J Am Acad Child Adolesc Psychiatry. (2002). , 41, 1078-1085.

[69] Gutteling, B. M, Weerth, C, Willemsen-swinkels, S, et al. The effects of prenatal stress on temperament and problem behavior of 27-month-old toddlers. Eur Child Adoles Psy. (2005). , 14, 41-51.

[70] Jacobsen, T. Effects of postpartum disorders on parenting and on offspring. In: Miller LJ, ed. Postpartum Mood Disorders. Washington, DC: American Psychiatric Press; (1999)., 1999, 119-139.

[71] Neggers, Y, Goldenberg, R, Cliver, S, & Hauth, J. The relationship between psychosocial profile, health practices, and pregnancy outcomes. Acta Obstet Gynecol Scand. (2006)., 85(3), 277-285.

[72] Wen, S. W, Goldenberg, R. L, Cutter, G. R, Hoffman, H. J, & Cliver, S. P. Intrauterine growth retardation and preterm delivery: Prenatal risk factors in an indigent population. Am J Obstet Gynecol. (1990)., 162(1), 213-218.

[73] Zuckerman, B, Amaro, H, Bauchner, H, & Cabral, H. Depressive symptoms during pregnancy: Relationship to poor health behaviors. Am J Obstet Gynecol. (1989)., 160, 1107-1111.

[74] Gyllstrom, M, Hellerstedt, W. L, & Hennrikus, D. The association of maternal mental health with prenatal smoking cessation and postpartum relapse in a population-based sample. Matern Child Health J. (2012)., 16(3), 685-693.

[75] Zhu, S, & Valbo, A. Depression and smoking during pregnancy. Addict Behav. (2002)., 27, 649-658.

[76] Ludman, E. J, Mcbride, C. M, Nelson, J. C, Curry, S. J, & Grothaus, L. C. Stress, depression and smoking cessation among pregnant women. Health Psychology. (2000)., 19, 1-8.

[77] Goedhart, G, Van Der Wal, M. F, Cuijpers, P, & Bonsel, G. J. Psychosocial problems and continued smoking during pregnancy. Addictive Behaviors. (2009)., 34(4), 403-406.

[78] Hobel, C. J. Stress and preterm birth. Clin Obstet Gynecol. (2004)., 47(4), 856-880.

[79] Chrousos, G. P, Torpy, D. J, & Gold, P. W. Interactions between the hypothalamic-pituitaryadrenal axis and the female reproductive system: clinical implications. Ann Intern Med. (1998)., 129, 229-240.

[80] Chrousos, G. P. The HPA axis and the stress response. Endocr Res. (2000)., 26, 513-4.

[81] Mcewen, B. Physiology and neurobiology of stress and adaptation: Central role of the brain. Physiol Rev. (2007)., 87, 873-904.

[82] Lu, M. C, & Halfon, N. Racial and ethnic disparities in birth outcomes: A life-course perspective. Matern Child Health J. (2003)., 7, 13-32.

[83] Wadhwa, P. D, Entringer, S, Buss, C, & Lu, M. C. The contribution of maternal stress to preterm birth: Issues and considerations. Clin Perinatol. (2011)., 38, 351-384.

[84] Chrousos, G. P, & Gold, P. W. The concepts of stress and stress system disorders. Overview of physical and behavioral homeostasis. JAMA. (1992)., 267, 1244-1252.

[85] Holzman, C, Jetton, J, Siler-khodr, T, et al. Second trimester corticotropin-releasing hormone levels in relation to preterm delivery and ethnicity. Obstet Gynecol. (2001)., 97, 657-663.

[86] Yanovski, J. A, Yanovski, S. Z, Friedman, T. C, et al. Etiology of the differences in corticotropin-releasing hormone-induced adrenocorticotropin secretion of black and white women. J Clin Endocrinol Metab. (1996)., 81, 3307-3311.

[87] Arck, P. C. Stress and pregnancy loss: role of immune mediators, hormones and neurotransmitters. Am J Reprod Immunol. (2001).

[88] Mastorakos, G, & Ilias, I. Maternal hypothalamic-pituitary adrenal axis in pregnancy and the postpartum period. Postpartum-related disorders. Ann NY Acad Sci. (2000)., 900, 95-106.

[89] Etringer, S, Buss, C, & Wadhwa, P. D. Prenatal stress and developmental programming of human health and disease risk: Concepts and integration of empirical findings. Curr Opin Endocrinol Diabetes Obes. (2010)., 17(6), 507-516.

[90] Mesiano, S, & Jaffe, R. B. Developmental and functional biology of the primate fetal adrenal cortex. Endocrine Reviews. (1997)., 18(3), 378-403.

[91] Smith, R, Mesiano, S, Chan, E. C, et al. Corticotropin-releasing hormone directly and preferentially stimulates dehydroepiandrosterone sulfate secretion by human fetal adrenal cortical cells. J Clin Endocrinol Metab. (1998)., 83, 2916-2920.

[92] Smith, R, Smith, J. I, Xiaobin, S, et al. Patterns of plasma corticotropin-releasing hormone, progesterone, estradiol, and estriol change and the onset of human labor. J Clin Endocrinol Metab. (2009)., 94, 2066-2074.

[93] Torche, F. The effect of maternal stress on birth outcomes: exploiting a natural experiment. Demography. (2011).

[94] Mclean, M, Bisits, A, Davies, J, Woods, R, Lowry, P, & Smith, R. A placental clock controlling the length of human pregnancy. Nat Med. (1995)., 1(5), 460-463.

[95] Mclean, M. Smith R: Corticotropin-releasing hormone in human pregnancy and parturition. Trends Endocrinol Metab. (1999)., 10, 174-178.

[96] Batemann, A, Singh, A, & Kral, T. Solomon S: The immune-hypothalamic-pituitary-adrenal axis. Endoc Rev. (1989)., 10, 92-102.

[97] Cupps, T. R. Fauci AS: Corticosteroid-mediated immunoregulation in man. Immun Rev. (1982)., 65, 133-155.

[98] Homo-delarche, F. Glucocorticoids, lymphokines and cell response. In Progress in Endocrinology, H Imura (ed.), Amsterdam, Elsevier, (1988)., 349-354.

[99] Rozanski, A, Blumenthal, J. A, Davidson, K. W, Saab, P. G, & Kubzansky, L. The epidemiology, pathophysiology, and management of psychosocial risk factors in

cardiac practice: The emerging field of behavioral cardiology. J Am Coll Cardiol. (2005). , 45, 637-651.

[100] Nicholson, A, Fuhrer, R, & Marmot, M. Psychological distress as a predictor of CHD events in men: the effect of persistence and components of risk. Psychosom Med. (2005).

[101] Esler, M, Schwarz, R, & Alvarenga, M. Mental stress is a cause of cardiovascular diseases: from scepticism to certainty. Stress Health. (2008). , 24, 175-180.

[102] Kyrou, I, Chrousos, G. P, & Tsigos, C. Stress, visceral obesity, and metabolic complications. Ann N Y Acad Sci. (2006).

[103] Ruiz, R. J, Fullerton, J, Brown, C. E, & Dudley, D. J. Predicting risk of preterm birth: The roles of stress, clinical risk factors, and corticotropin-releasing hormone. Biol Res Nurs. (2002). , 4, 54-64.

[104] Black, P. H. The inflammatory response is an integral part of the stress response: Implications for atherosclerosis, insulin resistance, type II diabetes and metabolic syndrome X. Brain Behav Immun. (2003). , 17, 350-364.

[105] Shurin, M. R, Lu, L, Kalinski, P, Stewart-akers, A. M, & Lotze, M. T. Th1/Th2 balance in cancer, transplantation and pregnancy. Immunopathol. (1999). , 21, 339-3359.

[106] Krishnan, L, Guilbert, L, Russell, A. S, Wegmann, T. G, & Mosmann, T. R. Belosevic M: Pregnancy impairs resistance of C57BL/6 mice to Leishmania major infection and causes decreased antigen-specific IFN-gamma response and increased production of T helper 2 cytokines. J Immunol. (1996). , 156, 644-652.

[107] Clark, D. A, Chaouat, G, Arck, P. C, & Mittruecker, H. W. Levy GA: Cytokine-dependent abortion in CBA×DBA/2 mice is mediated by the procoagulant fgl2 prothrombinase. J Immunol. (1998). , 160, 545-549.

[108] Clark, D. A, Ding, J. W, & Chaouat, G. Levy GA: The emerging role of immunoregulation of fibrinogen-related procoagulant Fgl2 in the success or spontaneous abortion of early pregnancy in mice and humans. Am J Reprod Immunol. (1999). , 42, 37-43.

[109] Silver, R. M, Lohner, W. S, Daynes, R. A, Mitchell, M. D, & Branch, D. W. Lipopolysaccharide-induced fetal death: The role of tumor-necrosis factor? Biol Reprod. (1994). , 50, 1108-1114.

[110] Arck, P. C, Merali, F. S, Manuel, J, Chaouat, G, & Clark, D. A. Stress-triggered abortion: inhibition of protective suppression and promotion of tumor necrosis factor (TNF) release as a mechanism triggering resorptions in mice. Am J Reprod Immunol. (1995). , 33, 74-80.

[111] Goldenberg, R. L, Hauth, J. C, & Andrews, W. W. Intrauterine infection and preterm delivery. New Engl J Med. (2000). , 342, 1500-1507.

[112] Sapolsky, R. M. Social subordinance as a marker of hypercortisolism: Some unexpected subtleties. Ann NY Acad Sci. (1995). , 771, 626-39.

[113] Kristenson, M, Kucinskien, Z, Bergdahl, B, Calkauskas, H, Urmonas, V, & Orth-gomer, K. Increased psychosocial strain in Lithuanian versus Swedish men: The Livicorida study. Psychosom Med (1998)., 60, 277-82.

[114] Geronimus, A. T. Black/white differences in the relationship of maternal age to birthweight: A population-based test of the weathering hypothesis. Soc Sci Med. (1996)., 42(4), 589-597.

[115] Noll, J. G, Schulkin, J, Trickertt, P. K, et al. Differential pathways to preterm delivery for sexually abused and comparison women. J Pediatr Psychol. (2007). , 32(10), 1238-1248.

[116] Love, C, David, R. J, Rankin, K. M, & Collins, J. W. Exploring weathering: Effects of lifelong economic environment and maternal age on low birth weight, small for gestational age, and preterm birth in African-American and white women. Am J Epidemiol. (2010)., 172(2), 127-134.

[117] Carpenter, L. L, Tyrka, A. R, Mcdougle, C. J, et al. Cerebrospinal fluid corticotropin-releasing factor and perceived early-life stress in depressed patients and healthy control subjects. Neuropsychopharmacol. (2004)., 29(4), 777-784.

[118] Elzinga, B. M, Roelofs, K, Tollenaar, M. S, Bakvis, P, Van Pelt, J, & Spinhoven, P. Diminished cortisol responses to psychosocial stress associated with lifetime adverse events a study among healthy young subjects. Psychoneuroendocrino. (2008)., 33(2), 227-237.

[119] Gonzalez, A, Jenkins, J. M, Steiner, M, & Fleming, A. S. The relation between early life adversity, cortisol awakening response and diurnal salivary cortisol levels in postpar tum women. Psychoneuroendocrino. (2009)., 34(1), 76-86.

[120] Shea, A. K, Streiner, D. L, Fleming, A, Kamath, M. V, Broad, K, & Steiner, M. The effect of depression, anxiety and early life trauma on the cortisol awakening response during pregnancy: Preliminary results. Psychoneuroendocrino. (2007)., 32, 1013-1020.

[121] Hazel, N. A, Hammen, C, Brennan, P. A, & Najman, J. Early childhood adversity and adolescent depression: The mediating role of continued stress. Psychol Med. (2008)., 38(4), 581-589.

[122] Seedat, S, Stein, D. J, Jackson, P. B, Heeringa, S. G, Williams, D. R, & Myer, L. Life stress and mental disorders in the South African stress and health study. SAMJ S Afr Med J. (2009)., 99, 375-382.

[123] Danese, A, Moffitt, T, Harrington, H, et al. Adverse childhood experiences and adult risk factors for age-related disease: Depression, inflammation, and clustering of metabolic risk markers. Arch Pediat Adolesc Med. (2009).

[124] DiPietro JAThe role of prenatal maternal stress in child development. Curr Dir Psychol Sci. (2004)., 13, 71-74.

[125] Kingston, D, Sword, W, Krueger, P, Hanna, S, & Markle-reid, M. Life course pathways to prenatal maternal stress. JOGNN. (2012). , 00, 1-18.

[126] Yali, A. M, & Lobel, M. Coping and distress in pregnancy: an investigation of medically high risk women. J Psychosom Obst Gyn. (1999).

[127] Lynn, F. A, Alderdice, F. A, Crealey, G. E, & Mcelnay, J. C. Associations between maternal characteristics and pregnancy-related stress among low-risk mothers: An observational cross-sectional study. Int J Nurs Stud. (2011). , 48, 620-627.

[128] Dunkel Schetter CLobel M. Pregnancy and birth: A multilevel analysis of stress and birth weight. In: Baum A, Revenson A, Singer J, eds. Handbook of Health Psychology. 2nd ed. New York, NY: Psychology Press;(2012).

[129] Barker, D, & Osmond, C. Infant mortality, childhood nutrition, and ischaemic heart disease in England and Wales. Lancet. (1986). , 1, 1077-1081.

[130] Barker, D, Winter, P, Osmond, C, Margetts, B, & Simmonds, S. Weight in infancy and death from ischaemic heart disease. Lancet. (1989). , 2, 577-580.

[131] Barker, D. J, Osmond, C, Simmonds, S. J, & Wield, G. A. The relation of small head circumference and thinness at birth to death from cardiovascular disease in adult life. Brit Med J. (1993).

[132] Spalding, D. A. Instinct with original observation on young animals. Br J Animal Behav. (1954).

[133] Hahn, P. Effect of litter size on plasma cholesterol and insulin and some liver and adipose tissue enzymes in adult rodents. J Nutr. (1984).

[134] Mott, G. E, Lewis, D. S, & Mcgill, H. C. Programming of cholesterol metabolism by breast or formula feeding. In: Bock GR, Whelan J, ed. The childhood environment and adult disease. Chichester: Wiley, (1991). CIBA Foundation Symposium 156.)

[135] Dobbing, J. Nutritional growth restriction and the nervous system. In: Davison AN, Thompson RHS, eds. The molecular bases of neuropathology. London: Edward Arnold, (1981).

[136] Smart, J. Undernutrition, learning and memory: review of experimental studies. In: Taylor TG, Jenkins NK, eds. Proceedings of XII international congress of nutrition. London: John Libbey, (1986).

[137] Lumey, L. H, & Stein, A. D. Offspring birth weights after maternal intrauterine undernutrition: A comparison within sibships. Am J Epidemiol. (1997). , 146, 810-820.

[138] Gluckman, P. D, Hanson, M. A, Spencer, H. G, & Bateson, P. Environmental influences during development and their later consequences for health and disease: Implications for the interpretation of empirical studies. P Roy Soc B-Biol Sci. (2005). , 272, 671-677.

[139] Bateson, P, Barker, D, Clutton-brock, T, et al. Developmental plasticity and human health. Nature. (2004).

[140] Connor, O, Heron, T. G, Golding, J, & Glover, J. V. Maternal antenatal anxiety and behavioural/emotional problems in children: A test of a programming hypothesis. J Child Psychol Psych. (2003).

[141] Deave, T, Heron, J, Evans, J, & Emond, A. The impact of maternal depression in pregnancy on early child development. Brit J Obstet Gynaec. (2008).

[142] Laplante, D. P, Brunet, A, Schmitz, N, Ciampi, A, & King, S. Project Ice Storm: Prenatal Maternal Stress Affects Cognitive and Linguistic Functioning in 5½-Year-Old Children. J Am Acad Child Psy. (2008). , 47, 1063-1072.

[143] Bergman, K, Sarkar, P, Connor, O, Modi, T. G, & Glover, N. V. Maternal stress during pregnancy predicts cognitive ability and fearfulness in infancy. J Am Acad Child Psy. (2007).

[144] Schneider, M. L, & Moore, C. F. Effect of prenatal stress on development: A nonhuman primate model. In: Nelson C, ed. The Effects of Early Adversity on Neurobehavioral Development. Mahwah, NJ: Erlbaum; (2000). , 2000, 201-243.

[145] Coe, C. L, & Lubach, G. R. Fetal Programming: Prenatal origins of health and illness. Curr Dir Psychol Sci. (2008). , 17, 36-41.

[146] Weaver, I. C, Champagne, F. A, Brown, S. E, et al. Reversal of maternal programming of stress responses in adult offspring through methyl supplementation: Altering epigenetic marking later in life. J Neurosci. (2005). , 25(47), 11045-11054.

[147] Seckl, J. R. Physiologic programming of the fetus. Emerging Concepts in Perinatal endocrinology. (1998). , 25, 939-962.

[148] Soumi, S. J. Early determinants of behavior: Evidence form primate studies. Br Med Bull. (1997). , 53, 170-184.

[149] Mizoguchi, K, Ishige, A, Aburada, M, & Tabira, T. Chronic stress attenuates glucocorticoid negative feedback: Involvement of the prefrontal cortex and hippocampus. Neuroscience. (2003). , 119(3), 887-897.

[150] Charil, A, Laplante, D. P, Vaillancourt, C, & King, S. Prenatal stress and brain development. Brain Res Rev. (2010). , 65, 56-79.

[151] Field, T, Diego, M, Hernandez-reif, M, et al. Pregnancy anxiety and comorbid depression and anger: Effects on the fetus and neonate. Depress Anxiety. (2003). , 17, 140-151.

[152] Gutteling, B. M, Weerth, C, & Zandbelt, N. Mulder EJH, Visser GHA, Buitelaar JK. Does maternal prenatal stress adversely affect the child's learning and memory at age six? J Abnorm Child Psychol. (2006). , 34, 789-798.

[153] Epel, E. S, Blackburn, E. H, Lin, J, Dhabhar, F. S, Adler, N. E, Morrow, J. D, et al. Accelerated telomere shortening in response to life stress. Proc Natl Acad Sci USA. (2004). , 101, 17312-17315.

[154] Lynch, M. E, Johnson, K. C, Kable, J. A, et al. Smoking in pregnancy and parenting stress: Maternal psychological symptoms and socioeconomic status as potential mediating variables. Nicotine Tob Res. (2011). , 13, 532-539.

[155] Fernander, A, Moorman, G, & Azuoru, M. Race-related stress and smoking among pregnant African-American women. Acta Obstet Gynecol Scand. (2010).

[156] Epsy, K. A, Fang, H, Johnson, C, et al. Prenatal tobacco exposure: Developmental outcomes in the neonatal period. Dev Psychol. (2011).

[157] Kowal, C, Kuk, J, & Tamim, H. Characteristics of weight gain in pregnancy among Canadian women. Matern Child Health J. (2012). , 16, 668-676.

[158] Woods, S. M, Melville, J. L, Guo, Y, et al. Psychosocial stress during pregnancy. Am J Obstet Gynecol. (2010).

[159] Robinson, T. E, & Berridge, K. C. Addiction. Annu. Rev. Psychol. (2003). , 54, 25-53.

[160] Pohorecky, L. A. Stress and alcohol interaction: An update of human research. Alcohol Clin Exp Res. (2003). , 15(3), 438-459.

[161] Kasl, S. V, Chisholm, R. F, & Eskenazi, B. The impact of the accident at the Three Mile Island on the behavior and well-being of nuclear workers: Part II: Job tension, psychophysiological symptoms, and indices of distress. Am J Public Health. (1981). , 71(5), 484-495.

[162] Tomkins, S. S. Psychological model of smoking behavior. Am J Public Health N. (1966). , 56, 17-20.

[163] Leventhal, H, & Cleary, P. D. The smoking problem: A review of the research and theory in behavioral risk modification. Psychol. Bull. (1980). , 88, 370-405.

[164] Russell, J. A, & Mehrabian, A. The mediating role of emotions in alcohol use. J Stud Alcohol. (1975). , 36, 1508-1536.

[165] Marlatt, G. A, & Gordon, J. R. Relapse Prevention: Maintenance Strategies in the Treatment of Addictive Behaviors. New York: Guilford Press; (1985).

[166] Wills, T, & Shiffman, S. Coping and substance abuse: A conceptual framework. In: Shiffman S, Wills T, eds. Coping and Substance Use. Orlando, FL: Academic Press; (1985). , 3-24.

[167] Khantzian, E. J. The self-medication hypothesis of addictive disorders: Focus on heroin and cocaine dependence. Am J Psychiatry. (1985). , 142, 1259-1264.

[168] Baker, T. B, Piper, M. E, Mccarthy, D. E, Majeskie, M. R, & Fiore, M. C. Addiction motivation reformulated: An affective processing model of negative reinforcement. Psychol Rev. (2004). , 111, 33-51.

[169] Koob, G. F. Le Moal M. Drug abuse: Hedonic homeostatic dysregulation. Science. (1997). , 278, 52-58.

[170] Laird, L. D, Amer, M. M, Barnett, E. D, & Barnes, L. L. Muslim patients and health disparities in the UK and the US. Arch Dis Child. (2007).

[171] Doyal, L. The Political Economy of Health. London: Pluto Press, (1979).

[172] Conrad, P, & Kern, R. eds. The Sociology of Health and Illness: Critical Perspectives. New York: St Martin's Press, (1981).

[173] Breilh, J. Epidemiologia Economia Medicina y Politica. Mexico City, Mexico: Distribuciones Fontamara, (1988). th edition; 1st edition published in 1979 by Universidad Central del Ecuador).

[174] Eyer, J, & Sterlin, P. Stress-related mortality and social organization. Rev Radical Pol Econ. (1977). , 9, 1-44.

[175] Navarro, V. Crisis, Health, and Medicine: A Social Critique. New York: Tavistock, (1986).

[176] Tesh, S. N. Hidden Arguments: Political Ideology and Disease Prevention Policy. New Brunswick, NJ: Rutgers University Press, (1988).

[177] Sanders, D. The Struggle for Health: Medicine and the Politics of Underdevelopment. Houndsmill, Basingstoke, Hampshire, and London: Macmillan, (1985).

[178] Turshen, M. The Politics of Public Health. New Brunswick, NJ: Rutgers University Press, (1989).

[179] Krieger, N. Theories for social epidemiology in the 21st century: An ecosocial perspective. Int J Epidemiol. (2001). , 30, 668 677.

[180] Link, B. G, & Phelan, J. C. Editorial: understanding sociodemographic differences in health- the role of fundamental social causes. Am J Public Health. (1996). , 86, 471-473.

[181] Dart, J. Australia's disturbing health disparities set Aboriginals apart. Bull World Health Organ. (2008). , 86, 245-247.

[182] Office for National StatisticsFocus on religion, (2001). Available at: http://www.ons.gov.uk/ons/rel/ethnicity/focus-on-religion/edition/index.html.Accessed July 31, 2012.

[183] Bukhari, Z. H. Demography, identity, space: defining American Muslims. In: Strum P, Tarantolo D, eds. Muslims in the United States. Washington, DC: Woodrow Wilson International Center for Scholars; (2003). , 2003, 7-21.

[184] Razzak, J. A, Khan, U. R, Azam, I, et al. Health disparities between Muslim and non-Muslim countries. East Mediterr Health J. (2011).

[185] Charasse-pouele, C, & Fournier, M. Health disparities between racial groups in South Africa: A decomposition analysis. Soc Sci Med. (2006). , 62, 2897-2914.

[186] Bradshaw, D, Matiseng, K, & Nannan, N. Health status and determinants. In: Ntuli A, Crisp N, Clarke E, Barron P, eds. South African health review 2000. Health System Trust, (2001).

[187] Burgard, S. Race and pregnancy-related care in Brazil and South Africa. Soc Sci Med. (2004). , 59(6), 1127-1146.

[188] Gennaro, S. Overview of current state of research on pregnancy outcomes in minority populations. Obstet Gynecol. (2005). SS10., 3.

[189] Centers for Disease Control and PreventionAchievements in public health, 1900-1999: healthier mothers and babies. MMWR Morb Mortal Wkly Rep. (1999). , 48, 849-58.

[190] Murphy, S. L, Xu, J, & Kochanek, K. D. Deaths: Preliminary data for 2010. National Vital Statistics Reports. (2012). , 60(4), 1-69.

[191] Centers for Disease Control and PreventionState-specific maternal mortality among black and white women: United States, 1987-1996. MMWR Morb Mortal Wkly Rep. (1999). , 48, 492-6.

[192] Demissie, K, Rhoads, G, Ananth, C, et al. Trends in preterm birth and neonatal mortality among blacks and whites in the United States from 1989 to 1997. Am J Epidemiol. (2001). , 154, 307-15.

[193] Lang, J, Lieberman, E, & Cohen, A. A comparison of risk factors for preterm labor and term small for gestational age birth. Epidemiology. (1996). , 7, 369-76.

[194] Malcoe, L, Shaw, G, Lammer, E, & Herman, A. The effect of congenital anomalies on mortality risk in white and black infants. Am J Public Health. (1999). , 89, 887-92.

[195] Zhang, H, & Bracken, M. Tree-based, two-stage risk factor analysis for spontaneous abortion. Am J Epidemiol. (1996). , 144, 989-96.

[196] Dorfman, S. Ectopic pregnancy surveillance. MMWR Morb Mortal Wkly Rep. (1983). , 32, 19-21.

[197] Barfield, W, Wise, P, Rust, F, Rist, K, Gould, J, & Gortmaker, S. Racial disparities in outcomes of military and civilian births in California. Arch Pediatr Adolesc Med. (1996). , 150, 1062-1067.

[198] Polednak, A. Black-white differences in infant mortality in 38 standard metropolitan statistical areas. Am J Public Health. (1991). , 81, 1480-2.

[199] Cabral, H, Fried, L. E, Levenson, S, Amaro, H, & Zuckerman, B. Foreign-born and US-born black women: differences in health behaviors and birth outcomes. Am J Public Health. (1990). e72.

[200] David, R, & Collins, J. Disparities in infant mortality: what's genetics got to do with it? Am J Pub Health. (2007). e1197.

[201] Dominguez, T. P. Race, racism, and racial disparities in adverse birth outcomes. Clin Obstet Gynecol. (2008). e370.

[202] Hogan, V. K, & Ferre, C. D. The social context of pregnancy for African American women: Implications for the study and prevention of adverse perinatal outcomes. Matern Child Healt J. (2001). , 5, 67-69.

[203] Feldman, P. Dunkel Schetter C, Woo G, Hobel CJ. Socioeconomic status and ethnicity in psychosocial processes during pregnancy. Ann Behav Med. (1997). S039.

[204] Krieger, N, Rowley, D, Herman, A. A, Avery, B, & Phillips, M. T. Racism, sexism, and social class: Implications for studies of health, disease, and well-being. Am J Prev Med. (1993). , 9, 82-122.

[205] Dominguez, T. Racial differences in birth outcomes. Health Psychol. (2008). , 27, 194-203.

[206] Ruiz, R. J, Fullerton, J, & Dudley, D. J. The interrelationship of maternal stress, endocrine factors and inflammation on gestational length. Obstet Gynecol Surv. (2003). , 58, 415-428.

[207] Mclafferty, S, & Tempalski, B. Restructuring and women's reproductive health: Implications for low birth weight in New York City. Geoforum. (1995). , 6, 309-323.

[208] Nkansah-amandra, S, Luchok, K. J, Hussey, J. R, Watkins, K, & Liu, X. Effects of maternal stress on low birth weight and preterm birth outcomes across neighborhoods of South Carolina, 2000-2003. Matern Child Health J. (2010). , 14, 215-226.

[209] Health Resources and Services AdministrationHealthy Start. Available at: http://mchb.hrsa.gov/programs/healthystart/index.html.Accessed May 17, (2012).

[210] Alderdice, F, Lynn, F, & Lobel, M. A review and psychometric evaluation of pregnancy-specific stress measures. J Psychosom Obst Gyn. (2012). , 33(2), 62-77.

[211] Goldberg, D. The Detection of Psychiatric Illness by Questionnaire: A Technique for the Identification and Assessment of Non-Psychotic Psychiatric Illness. London: Oxford University Press; (1972).

[212] Goldberg, D. P, & Williams, P. A User's Guide to the GHQ. Windsor, NFER-Nelson, (1988).

[213] Cook, M, Young, A, Taylor, D, & Bedford, A. Personality correlates of psychological distress. Pers Indiv Differ. (1996). , 20, 313-319.

[214] Ivkovic, V, Vitart, V, Rudan, I, et al. The Eysenck personality factors: Psychometric structure, reliability, heritability and phenotypic and genetic correlations with psychological distress in an isolated Croatian population. Pers Indiv Differ. (2007). , 42, 123-133.

[215] Ploubidis, G, Abbott, R, Huppert, F, Kuh, D, Wadsworth, M, & Croudace, T. Improvements in social functioning reported by a birth cohort in mid-adult life: A person-centered analysis of GHQ-28 social dysfunction items using latent class analysis. Pers Indiv Differ. (2007). , 42, 305-316.

[216] Jackson, C. The General Health Questionnaire. Occup Med-C. (2007).

[217] Alhamad, A, & Al-faris, E. A. The validation of the general health questionnaire (GHQ-28) in a primary care setting in Saudi Arabia. J Family Community Med. (1998)., 5(1), 13-19.

[218] Quek, K. F, Low, W. Y, Razack, A. H, & Loh, C. S. Reliability and validity of the General Health Questionnaire (GHQ-12) among urological patients: a Malaysian study. Psychiatry Clin Neurosci. (2001)., 55(5), 509-13.

[219] Werneke, U, Goldber, D. P, Yalcin, I, & Ustun, B. T. The stability of the factor structure of the General Health Questionnaire. Psychol Med. (2000)., 30, 823-829.

[220] Goldberg, D. P, Gater, R, Satorius, N, et al. The validity of two versions of the GHQ in the WHO study of mental illness in general health care. Psychol Med. (1997)., 27, 191-197.

[221] Cohen, S, Kamarck, T, & Mermelstein, R. A global measure of perceived stress. J Health Soc Behav. (1983)., 24(4), 385-396.

[222] Cohen, S, & Williamson, G. M. Perceived stress in a probability sample of the United States. In: Spacapan S, Oskamp S, eds. The Social Psychology of Health. Newbury Park, CA: Sage; (1988)., 1988, 31-67.

[223] Cole, S. R. Assessment of differential item functioning in the Perceived Stress Scale-10. J Epidemiol Community Health. (1999)., 53, 319-320.

[224] DiPietro JAHilton SC, Hawkins M, Costigan KA, Pressman EK. Maternal stress and affect influence fetal neurobehavioral development. Dev Psychol.(2002).

[225] Roesch, S. C. Dunkel Schetter C, Woo G, Hobel CJ. Modeling the types and timing of stress in pregnancy. Anxiety Stress Copin. (2004)., 17, 87-102.

[226] Hawkins, M. DiPietro JA, Costigan KA. Social class differences in maternal stress appraisal during pregnancy. Ann N Y Acad Sci. (1999)., 896, 439-441.

[227] Monk, C, Leight, K. L, & Fang, Y. The relationship between women's attachment style and perinatal mood disturbance: Implications for screening and treament. Arch Womens Ment Health. (2008)., 11, 117-129.

[228] Van den Bergh BRThe influence of maternal emotions during pregnancy on fetal and neonatal behavior. J Prenat Perinat Psychol Health. (1990)., 5, 119-130.

[229] Rini, C. K. Dunkel Schetter C, Wadhwa PD, Sandman CA. Psychological adaptation and birth outcomes: The role of personal resources, stress, and sociocultural context in pregnancy. Health Psychol. (1999).

[230] Mancuso, R. A, Schetter, C. D, Rini, C. M, Roesch, S. C, & Hobel, C. J. Maternal prenatal anxiety and corticotropin-releasing hormone associated with timing of delivery. Psychosom Med. (2004)., 66, 762-769.

[231] Dominguez, T. P, Schetter, C. D, Mancuso, R, Rini, C. M, & Hobel, C. Stress in African American pregnancies: Testing the roles of various stress concepts in prediction of birth outcomes. Ann Behav Med. (2005). , 29, 12-21.

[232] Gurung RARDunkel Schetter C, Collins N, Rini C, Hobel CJ. Psychosocial predictors of prenatal anxiety. J Soc Clin Psychol. (2005). , 24, 497-519.

[233] Alderdice, F, & Lynn, F. Factor structure of the prenatal distress questionnaire. Midwifery. (2011). , 27(4), 553-559.

[234] Lobel, M, Devincent, C. J, Kaminer, A, & Meyer, B. A. The impact of prenatal maternal stress and optimistic disposition on birth outcomes in medically high-risk women. Health Psychol. (2000). , 19, 544-553.

[235] Gennaro, S, Shults, J, & Garry, D. J. Stress and preterm labor and birth in Black women. J Obstet Gynecol Neonatal Nurs. (2008). , 37, 538-545.

[236] Pluess, M, Bolten, M, Pirke, K. M, & Hellhammer, D. Maternal trait anxiety, emotional distress, and salivary cortisol in pregnancy. Biol Psychol. (2010). , 83, 169-175.

[237] Orr, S. T, James, S. A, & Casper, R. Psychosocial stressors and low birth weight: Development of a questionnaire. J Dev Behav Pediatr. (1992). , 13, 343-347.

[238] Hulka, B. S. Overview of biological markers. In: Hulka BS, Griffith JD, Wilcosky TC, eds, Biological markers in epidemiology. New York: Oxford University Press; (1990). , 1990, 3-15.

[239] Obel, C, Hedegaard, M, Henriksen, T. B, Secher, N. J, Olsen, J, & Levine, S. Stress and salivary cortisol during pregnancy. Psychoneuroendocrino. (2005). , 30, 647-656.

[240] Giurgescu, C. Are maternal cortisol levels related to preterm birth? JOGNN. (2009). , 38, 377-390.

[241] Pitiphat, W, Gillman, M. W, Joshipura, K. J, Williams, P. L, Douglass, C. W, & Rich-edwards, J. W. Plasma c-reactive protein in early pregnancy and preterm delivery. Am J Epidemiol. (2005). , 162(11), 1108-1113.

[242] Nater, U. M, Rohleder, N, Gaab, J, et al. Human salivary alpha-amylase reactivity in a psychosocial stress paradigm. Int J Psychophysiol. (2005). , 55, 333-342.

[243] Mayeux, R. Biomarkers: Potential uses and limitations. NeuroRx. (2004). , 1, 182-188.

[244] Gordis, L. Epidemiology and public policy. In: Epidemiology (Gordis L, ed), Philadelphia: W.B. Saunders, (1996). , 247-256.

[245] Harville, E. W, Gunderson, E. P, Matthews, K. A, Lewis, C. E, & Carnethon, M. Pre-pregnancy stress reactivity and pregnancy outcome. Paediatr Perinat Epidemiol. (2010).

Chapter 3

The Role of the Coagulation System in Preterm Parturition

Vered Klaitman, Ruth Beer-Wiesel, Tal Rafaeli,
Moshe Mazor and Offer Erez

Additional information is available at the end of the chapter

http://dx.doi.org/10.5772/54843

1. Introduction

Term and preterm parturition have a common pathway that includes irregular uterine contractions, cervical effacement and dilatation, along with decidual activation and rupturing of the chorioamniotic membrane. This pathway is observed in the physiologic labor at term as well as in the pathological processes leading to premature delivery. Indeed, the clinical presentation of preterm parturition involves all components of this common pathway: 1. Preterm contractions in women with spontaneous preterm labor with intact membranes; 2.cervical effacement and dilatation in women with cervical insufficiency; and/or 3.decidual activation and rupture of membranes in those with preterm PROM.

The syndrome of preterm parturition is the clinical presentation of several underlying mechanisms, not all of them being fully understood. Among the well establishes etiologies for preterm parturition are: intra amniotic infection/inflammation, cervical insufficiency, increased thrombin generation and vascular pathology of the placenta, as well as multiple gestations. The study of the maternal fetal interface and the placenta contributes to the deciphering of the mechanism leading to preterm birth. Placental and decidual vascular lesions have been reported in about 20-30% of patients who deliver preterm. There are accumulating evidence that preterm parturition is associated with an increased activation of maternal hemostatic system which also interacts with the acute inflammatory processes observed in this syndrome. Moreover, higher rates of fetal growth restriction and placental vascular lesions were observed among women with preterm labor who delivered at term suggesting that some vascular insults may not be severe enough to cause preterm birth but still inflict some effect on fetal growth.

The following chapter will summarize the changes in maternal hemostatic system during normal pregnancy and those associated with preterm labor and preterm PROM. In addition, we will review the vascular changes associated with preterm parturition. The last section of this chapter will address the role of the hemostatic and angiogenic markers for the prediction of spontaneous preterm birth.

2. The physiology of hemostasis

Hemostasis is crucial for the maintenance of the vascular tree integrity.

The major components of the hemostatic system, which function in concert, are the following: 1) the vessel wall and endothelium; 2) platelets and other formed elements of blood, such as monocytes and red cells; and 3) plasma proteins (the coagulation and fibrinolytic factors and inhibitors). These components act altogether in a synchronize fashion to generate the hemostatic plug, preserve the integrity of the vascular tree in the body, and avoid uncontrolled clot formation and thrombosis (See figure 1).

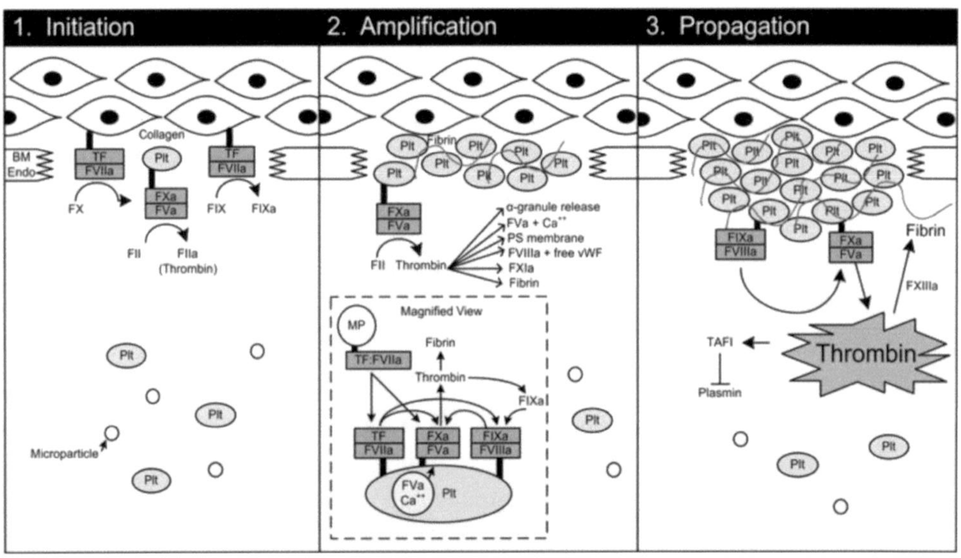

Figure 1. Initiation of coagulation by endothelial injury and exposure of tissue factor to the extrinsic pathway. Then, the platelets aggregate by activation of intrinsic pathway and platelet activation. And finally propagation and clot stabilization by thrombin – fibrin balance formation (from reference #12 with permission).

The vessel wall: Endothelial damage or activation is a crucial event that launches the cascade of reactions leading to thrombin generation and fibrin clot formation. The vascular endothelium is the focal point for both initiation and inhibition of the coagulation process. During endothelial damage the sub endothelial tissue factor molecules are exposed and initiate coagulation by activation of the extrinsic pathway. This is relevant also for the maternal fetal interface since the villous and exteravillos trophoblast of the human placenta adopt the properties of endothelium and vessel wall in order to allow laminar flow of maternal blood through the placental bed without unnecessary activation of the coagulation cascade; and any damage in their integrity will activate the coagulation cascade.

Platelets activation and plaque formation: Following vascular injury platelets initially adhere to sub-endothelial collagen via von Willebrand factor (vWF) (figure 2). These vWF "bridges" are anchored at one end to sub-endothelial type IV collagen molecules and at the other end to the platelet GPIb/IX/V receptor [1,2]. The adherent platelets can also attach to other sub-endothelial extracellular matrix proteins (e.g. laminin, fibronectin, and vitronectin) via cell-membrane bound integrins [3]. The binding of these receptors activates the platelets through calcium-dependent cytoskeletal changes.

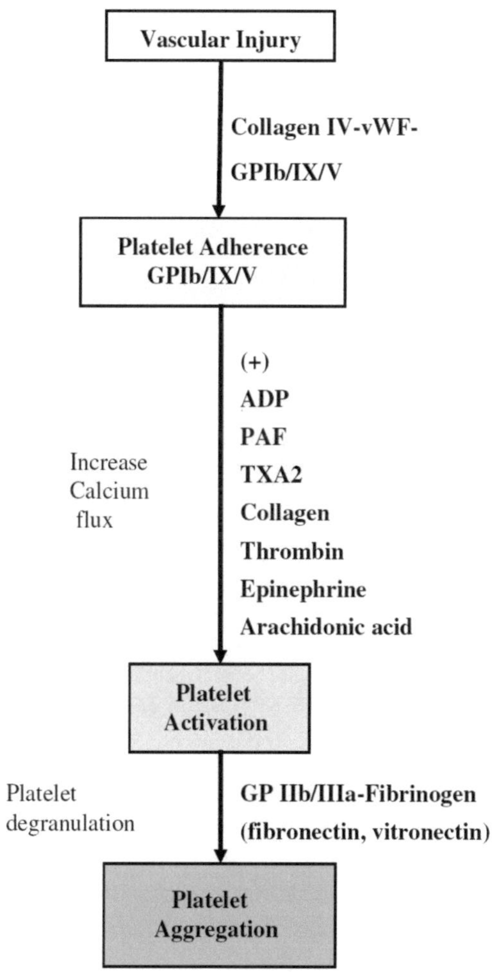

Figure 2. Mediators of platlet activation and agregation (from reference #5 with permission).

Activated platelets form pseudopodia that further enhance vWF coupling to the sub endothelium. Moreover, ADP induces a conformational change in the GPIIb/IIIa receptor on the platelet membrane causing platelet aggregation via the formation of a high affinity fibrinogen bridges anchored at either end by GPIIb/IIIa receptors on 2 different platelets [4]. Thus, Platelet activation converts the normally inactive Gp IIb/IIIa receptor into an active one, enabling binding to fibrinogen and VWF. Because the surface of each platelet has about 50,000 Gp IIb/IIIa-binding sites, numerous activated platelets recruited to the site of vascular injury can rapidly form an occlusive aggregate by means of a dense network of intercellular fibrinogen bridges. Since this receptor is the key mediator of platelet aggregation, it has become an effective target for antiplatelet therapy [5].

2.1. Plasma proteins

Coagulation factors: Plasma coagulation proteins (*clotting factors*) normally circulate in plasma in their inactive forms. The sequence of coagulation protein reactions that culminate in the formation of fibrin was originally described as a *waterfall* or a *cascade*. Two pathways of blood coagulation have been described in the past: the extrinsic, or tissue factor, pathway and the intrinsic or contact activation, pathway (figure 3). However, the current approach is a more unify view in which the coagulation cascade is normally initiated through tissue factor exposure and activation of the *extrinsic pathway* that generates thrombin and activates the elements of the classic *intrinsic pathway*. These reactions take place on phospholipid surfaces, usually on activated platelets.

The initial phase of coagulation is the exposure of tissue factor to coagulation factors, caused either by endothelial damage or activation [6]. Tissue factor (TF) is a 47kDa cell bound trans-membrane glycoprotein and member of class 2 cytokine superfamily [7], that functions as: 1) a receptor, with signal transduction resulting in the induction of genes involved in inflammation, apoptosis, embryonic development and cell migration[8]; and 2])as an activator and cofactor for factors VII/VIIa in the coagulation cascade. It is constitutively expressed by many extravascular tissues, especially perivascular ones, and it is highly expressed in the brain, heart, lungs, kidneys, testis and placenta [9-11], reflecting the importance of these tissues to the organism[12]. TF expression can be induced in monocytes and platelets, and has been detected on circulating microparticles (MP) derived from these and other cell types [7,13]. The expression of this coagulation factor can also be induced on endothelium in response to inflammatory stimuli including exposure to: 1) bacterial lipopolysaccharide (LPS) in sepsis; 2) adhesion molecules (P-selectin expressed on platelets, CD40 ligand expressed on white blood cells); and 3) inflammatory cytokines (interleukin- 6, tumor necrosis factor), and oxidized low-density lipoprotein(LDL) [14].

Tissue factor activates the coagulation cascade by binding to the serine protease factor VIIa; the complex of TF+FVIIa activates factor X to factor Xa and initiating the converting factor IX to factor IXa in the intrinsic system leading to further formation of factor Xa. Thus, this factor is formed through the actions of either the tissue factor/factor VIIa complex or factor IXa (with factor VIIIa as a cofactor), and converts pro-thrombin to thrombin, the pivotal protease of the coagulation system. Thrombin is a multifunctional enzyme that converts soluble plasma fibrinogen to an insoluble fibrin matrix. Thrombin also activates factor XIII (fibrin-stabilizing factor) to factor XIIIa, which covalently cross-links and thereby stabilizes the fibrin clot.

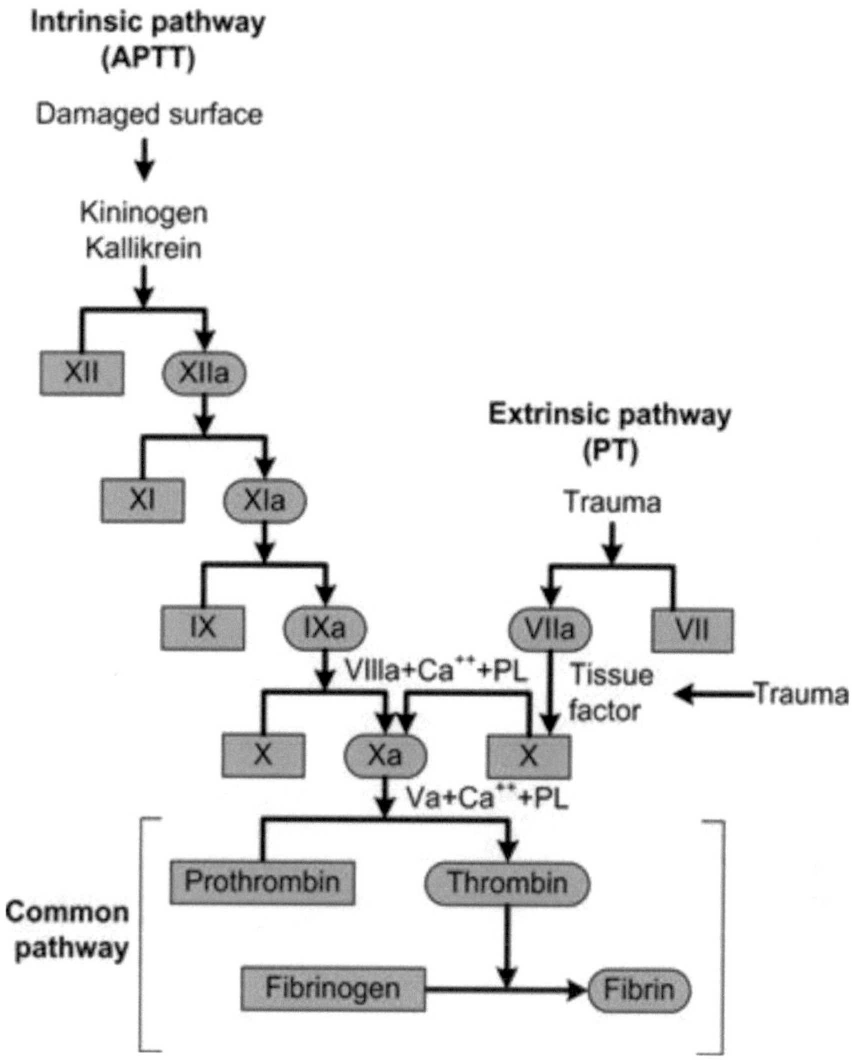

Figure 3. The extrinsic and intrinsic pathways of coagulation are a model for simplifying the coagulation system. This model is reflected in the laboratory PT and PTT measurements (from reference #12 with permission).

An additional mechanism in which the activation of the coagulation cascade can take place is through microparticles. Circulating microparticles are an area of intense research, as increased levels of them were shown to be pro-coagulant, even in the absence of TF expression [14-17]. These microparticles are tiny (<1 mm) membrane-bound vesicles and express membrane antigens that reflect their cellular origin[18]. The concentration of circulating microparticles is increased during platelet activation, inflammation, or apoptosis. Elevated concentrations of microparticles are encountered in diseases with vascular involvement and hypercoagulability such as disseminated intravascular coagulation, diabetes, and immune-mediated thrombosis [12].

Anti-coagulation protein:

Thrombin also plays a crucial role in activating the inhibition of the coagulation cascade.

Following its activation thrombin binds to thombomodulin causing a conformational change that activates the endothelial receptor of protein c, which in turns activates protein C. The latter is bound to its cofactor protein s together this complex inactivates factor Va and factor VIIIa of the intrinsic pathway, reducing substantially thrombin generation13. In addition to protein c and protein s there is the tissue factor pathway inhibitor (TFPI) which is the main inhibitor of the extrinsic pathway of coagulation, this protein inhibits the activity of factor VIIa and factor Xa reducing by this thrombin generation by the extrinsic pathway. the complex of protein z and Protein Z-dependent protease inhibitor (ZPI) inactivates factor Xa, and can also directly inhibit factor XIa. However, by far the most active inhibitor of both factor Xa and thrombin is antithrombin (AT) (previously known as antithrombin III). The AT molecule binds to either thrombin or factor Xa and then complexes with vitronectin which causes a conformational change that facilitates heparin binding. The resultant quaternary structure augments thrombin inactivation 1000-fold. The function of these anticoagulation protein is essential for maintaining the homeostasis between coagulation and adequate blood flow in the vascular tree, and deficiency in these protein is associated with increase risk for thromboembolic diseases and other complications.

Fibrinolysis factors and inhibitors: The process of fibrinolysis (i.e., clot lysis) is also crucial to the prevention of thrombosis (Figure 4). Fibrin is degraded to its degradation products (FDPs) by plasmin [19], that is generated from plasminogen by the action of tissue-type plasminogen activator (tPA) embedded in fibrin. This process is accelerated when plasminogen itself is bound to fibrin. Endothelial cells produce a second plasminogen activator, urokinase-type plasminogen activator (uPA). The latter's activation requires high molecular weight kininogen, kallikrein, and plasmin. This helps explain why deficiency of the former two "intrinsic pathway" clotting factors (ie, activators of factor XI) paradoxically lead to thrombosis and not bleeding.

There are series of inhibitors of premature fibrinolysis and, thus, hemorrhage. Plasmin is directly inhibited by a2-plasmin inhibitor. This inhibitor is also bound to the fibrin clot where it is positioned to prevent premature fibrinolysis. Type-1 plasminogen activator inhibitor (PAI-1) is synthesized by endothelial cells and platelets in response to thrombin binding to (protease activated receptor) PARs. In pregnancy, the decidua is a rich source of PAI-1, while the placenta produces PAI-1 and PAI -2, and serve as the primary source for the latter [20,21]. In the initial stages of platelet plug and fibrin clot formation, endothelial cells release PAI-1 but after a delay, endothelial cells release tPA and uPA to promote fibrinolysis.

Thrombin-activatable fibrinolysis inhibitor (TAFI) is another antifibrinolytic factor which acts by cleaving the C-terminal lysine in fibrin, to render it resistant to cleavage by plasmin [22,23]. Levels of TAFI are increased in the third trimester [23]. Interestingly, TAFI is also activated by the thrombin-thrombomodulin complex, once again implicating thrombin as the ultimate arbiter of hemostasis. The fibrinolytic system can influence coagulation in several ways. For example, FDPs inhibit thrombin action, a major source of hemorrhage in disseminated intravascular coagulation. In addition, PAI-1 bounded to vitronectin and also to heparin can directly inhibit thrombin and factor Xa activity [5,24].

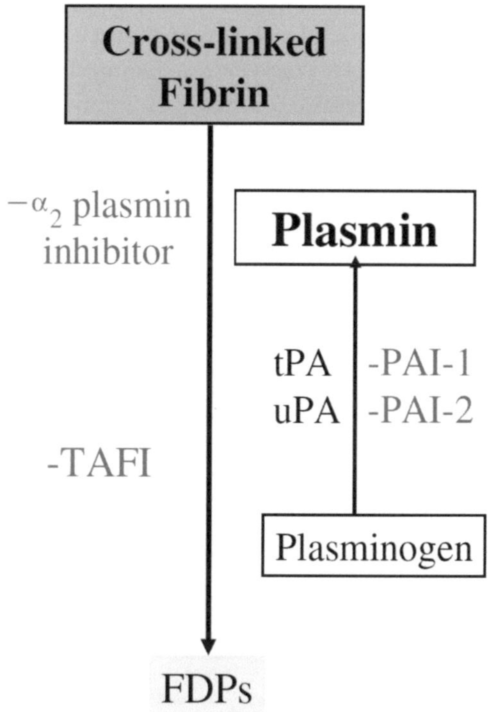

Figure 4. Fibrinolysis factors and inhibitors. The following scheme shows the process of fibrin degradation and plasmin generation (from reference #5 with permission).

3. Pregnancy associated changes in the hemostatic system

Pregnancy is a challenging time period for the hemostatic system. The demands from this system changes in different sites and are somewhat contradictory. The formation of the placental bed in which the maternal blood is running outside the maternal vessels necessitate the mother to address two challenges, the first one is to protect herself from a life threatening bleeding, and the second is to enable a continues blood flow through the placental bed outside the maternal blood vessels without activating the coagulation cascade. These challenges have been addressed by the formation of three compartments: 1) The maternal compartment which becomes adaptive and pro-coagulant to prevent severe bleeding during delivery; 2) The fetus that develops his coagulation system during gestation while floating in the pro-coagulant amniotic fluid; and 3) The maternal fetal interface of which the intervillous space is hypocoagulated in order to ensure the extravascular laminar flow of maternal blood and the maternal decidua is rich with tissue factor to prevent bleeding.

During gestation, changes in the coagulation system are considered to be adaptive to prevent hemorrhage at the time of delivery [25-29]. Indeed, normal pregnancy has been associated with excessive maternal thrombin generation [28,30] and a tendency for platelets to aggregate in response to agonists [31,32] (TABLE 1). Pregnancy is accompanied by 2 to 3-fold increase in fibrinogen concentrations and 20% to 1000% increase in factors VII, VIII, IX, X, and XII, all of which peak at term [33]. The concentrations of vWF increase up to 400% by term [33]. By contrast, those of pro-thrombin and factor V remain unchanged while the concentrations of factors XIII and XI decline modestly[34]. Indeed there is evidence of chronic low-level thrombin and fibrin generation throughout normal pregnancy as indicated by enhanced concentrations of pro-thrombin fragment 1.2, thrombin-antithrombin (TAT III) complexes, and soluble fibrin polymers[23]. Free protein S concentration declines significantly (up to 55%) during pregnancy due to increased circulating complement 4B-binding protein its molecular carrier. Protein S nadir at delivery and this reduction is exacerbated by cesarean delivery and infection [33,35]. As a consequence, pregnancy is associated with an increase in resistance to activated protein C [23,33]. The concentrations of PAI-1 increase by 3 to 4-folds during pregnancy while plasma PAI-2 values, which are negligible before pregnancy reach concentrations of 160 mg/L at delivery [33]. Thus, pregnancy is associated with increased clotting potential, as well as decreased anticoagulant properties, and fibrinolysis [5]. Therefore, it can be defined as a prothrombotic state.

		Increased	**Decreased**	**No change**
Systemic changes	Procoagulant factors	I,V,VII,VIII,IX,X	XI	
	Anticoagulant factors	Soluble TM	PS	
	Adhesive proteins	vWF		
	Fibrinolytic proteins	PAI-1,PAI-2	t-PA	TAFI
	Microparticles and APLA	MP		APLA
Local placental changes		TF	TFPI	

Table 1. Hemostatic changes in pregnancy [42].

In contrast to the maternal circulation and the decidua, the establishment of the uteroplacental circulation challenges the hemostatic system. Indeed, fibrin deposition sites were identified in decidual veins at sites of trophoblast invasion, where villi are implanted into veins [36]. Compared with endothelial vasculature, the trophoblasts lining decidual spiral arteries have a reduced capacity to lyse fibrin, and recent studies have shown that this is caused by high concentrations of plasminogen activator inhibitors [37] that affects it fybrinolytic capabilities. In addition, perivascular decidualized human endometrial stromal cells are ideally positioned to prevent postimplantation haemorrhage during endovascular trophoblast invasion by expressing TF, which is a primary cellular mediator of hemostasis [38,39]. In vivo and in vitro studies have demonstrated that estradiol (E2) enhances TF expression during progesterone induced decidualization. It was demonstrated that paracrine factors, such as endothelial growth factor (EGF) are involved with steroid-enhancing TF expression in decidualized human endometrial stromal cells through the EGF receptor [40]. The trophoblast and the placenta have distinct anticoagulation properties that aimed on one hand to prevent bleeding and on the other hand to allow laminar flow of maternal blood through the intervillous space [41,42]. Accumulating evidence suggest that the trophoblast acquires properties of vascular epithelium and expresses coagulation inhibitors such as tissue factor pathway inhibitor 2[43-45] (also known as placental protein 5 [46,47]), heparin co-factor II, dermatan sulfate [48, 49], and thrombomodulin [50-53] as well as pro-coagulant proteins such as tissue factor [38,54]. Moreover, a knockout mouse model for the endothelial receptor of protein C was lethal in-utero and the embryos died on the 10.5 day of gestation, and fibrin deposition was found around their giant trophoblast cells of these embryos [55]. Moreover, a recent report demonstrated that the placenta is an extra-hepatic source of the anti-coagulant proteins including protein C, protein S, as well as protein Z, and their expression is constitutive irrespective of obstetrical conditions [85].

4. The hemostatic system and preterm parturition

The involvement of the hemostatic system in the pathophysiology of preterm parturition is becoming more and more apparent. Indeed, changes in maternal and fetal gens, abnormal placental vascular finding and increased thrombin generation in the maternal circulation were all reported in association with preterm parturition.

Genetic studies: During parturition there is remodeling of the extra cellular matrix of the uterine cervix. Recently increased expression of the tissue type plasminogen activator gene was reported during labor at term [56]. This finding was supported by the role of plasminogen activation in the remodeling of the extracellular matrix in human amnion, chorio-decidua, and placenta during and after labor [57]. Moreover, in a genetic association study that tested maternal and fetal genes in women with preterm labor reported this gene to be highly express in fetuses of Hispanic patients who delivered preterm.

Single nucleotide polymorphisms of the coagulation genes are associated with increased risk for preterm birth. Indeed, in a study that aimed to identify the impact of genetic polymorphisms with pro-thrombotic and anti-thrombotic effects on the occurrence of preterm birth in a large cohort of very-low-birth-weight (VLBW)-infants and their mothers, and term-born-infants and their mothers, maternal factor VII-121del/ins and the infant's factor VII-121del/ins polymorphisms were more frequent in the group of singleton VLBW and their mothers. Furthermore, the frequency of the factor XIII-Val34Leu polymorphism was significantly lower in singleton VLBW than in term infant controls; and in a multivariate regression analysis, previous preterm delivery, the maternal carrier status of the factor-VII-121del/ins polymorphism (OR=1.7, 95% CI: 1.12-2.5, p=0.007) and the lower frequency of infant's factor-XIII-Val34Leu polymorphism (OR=0.53; 95% CI: 0.29-0.96; p=0.038) were found to be independently associated with preterm delivery [58]. The association between Polymorphisms in factor VII and preterm birth was also reported among Caucasian in the USA. This study included maternal and fetal DNA from 370 patients. For maternal data the strongest associations were found in genes in the complement-coagulation pathway related to decidual hemorrhage in preterm birth. In this pathway 3 of 6 genes examined had SNPs significantly associated with preterm birth, including factor V, factor VII, and tissue plasminogen activator. The single strongest effect was observed in tPA marker rs879293 with a significant allelic and genotypic association with preterm delivery (OR- 2.80, CI 1.77–4.44, for a recessive model). Finally, exploratory multi-locus analyses in the complement and coagulation pathway were performed and revealed a potentially significant interaction between a marker in Factor V (rs2187952) and Factor VII (rs3211719) (p<0.001); the authors concluded that "These results support a role for genes in both the coagulation and inflammation pathways, and potentially different maternal and fetal genetic risks for preterm birth"[59].

Collectively the evidence brought here suggest that genetic polymorphism of the coagulation genes may predispose a subset of women to an increased risk for preterm birth. What is the role of gene environmental interaction and in what mechanisms these polymorphisms of the coagulation genes affect the risk for preterm parturition are still unknown and are an area of future research.

Changes in maternal circulation: Increased thrombin generation in the maternal circulation, above that reported during normal pregnancy, has been reported in all the great obstetrical syndromes including preeclampsia [60-66], fetal growth restriction [61,62,67,68], fetal death [69], preterm labor (PTL) [30,70], and preterm PROM [30,69,71]. There are several possible explanations for the increased thrombin generation reported in women with preterm parturition: 1) increased activation of coagulation cascade in the maternal circulation due to pathological processes including bleeding or inflammation; and 2) depletion of anticoagulation proteins that subsequently leads to increased thrombin generation.

Increased activation of the coagulation cascade among women with preterm parturition is well supported by the current literature. Indeed, women with preterm PROM and preterm labor have a higher median maternal plasma concentration of thrombin-anti-thrombin (TAT) III complexes [30,70]. In addition, in women with preterm labor elevated maternal plasma TAT III concentration was associated with a higher chance to deliver within <7 days from admission [69] (figure 5, and figure 6). Median maternal plasma Tissue factor, concentration is higher in women with preterm PROM, but not in those with PTL, than in those with normal pregnancies [72]. Nevertheless, women with preterm labor as well as those with preterm PROM had both increased tissue factor activity in comparison to normal pregnant women.

http://dx.doi.org/10.5772/54843

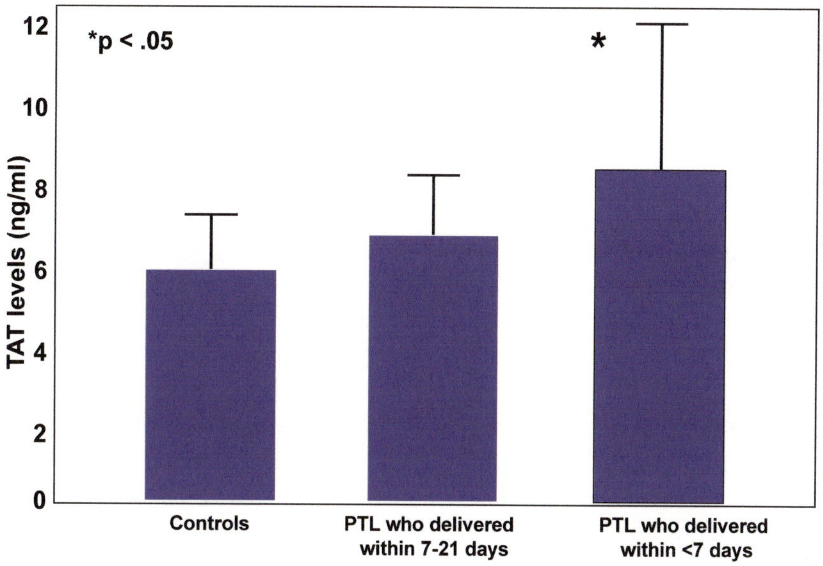

Figure 5. Thrombin–antithrombin III (*TAT*) levels in control patients, patients with preterm labor who delivered within 3 weeks, and patients with preterm labor who delivered after 3 weeks. *Open diamonds,* Mean levels; *black error bars,* SD. *P <.05, Student-Newman-Keuls method (from reference #70 with permission).

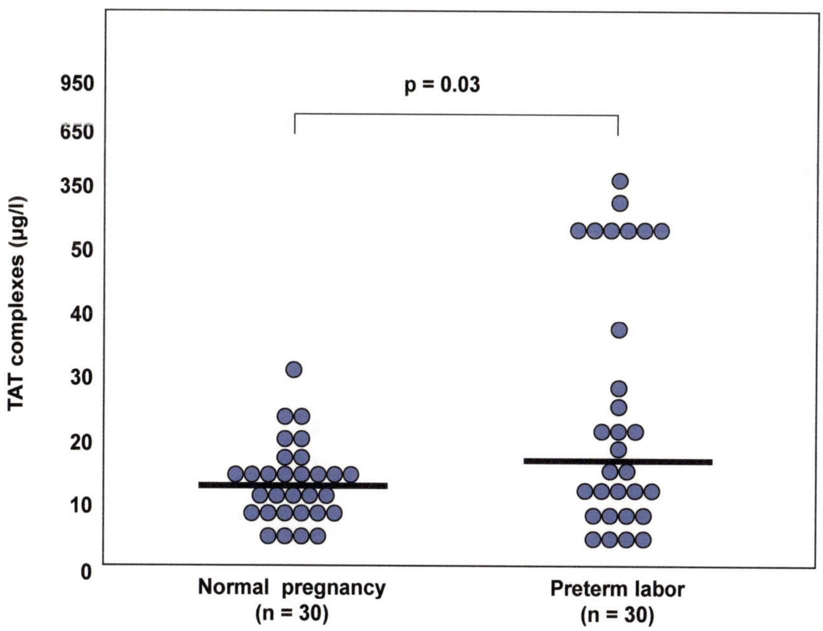

Figure 6. Maternal plasma TAT III concentration in women with preterm labor (PTL) and those with a Normal pregnancy (from reference #30 with permission).

The activation of the coagulation system in the placental and maternal compartment of patients with preterm parturition can result from the following underlying mechanisms: 1(decidual hemorrhage that leads to a retro-placental clot formation [73]; 2) intra-amniotic infection which can induce decidual bleeding and sub-clinical abruption [74], as well as increased intra-amniotic TAT complexes [69]; and 3) an increased maternal systemic inflammatory response [75] that may activate the extrinsic pathway of coagulation due to the expression and release of tissue factor (TF) by activated monocytes [76]. These mechanisms result in an increased thrombin generation, which has been associated with the following: 1) stimulation of decidual cell secretion of matrix metalloproteinase (MMP) (i.e. MMP-1 and MMP-3) that can degrade the extracellular matrix of the chorioamniotic membranes [77,78](as is in preterm PROM); and 2) myometrial activation and uterine contractions generation that may lead to preterm labor with or without rupture of membranes and a subsequent preterm delivery [70,79,80]. While thrombin is generated as a consequence of activation of the coagulation cascade, TF, the most powerful natural pro-coagulant, is abundant in the uterine decidua in the normal state [81,82], as part of an efficient hemostatic mechanism in the uterine wall, which is activated in the course of normal pregnancy during implantation[83] and after delivery[84]. However, this hemostatic mechanism may also be activated due to pathological decidual bleeding in pregnancies complicated by placental abruption [73,85] and intra-amniotic infection [74].

A novel mechanism that may lead to an increased thrombin generation in women with preterm parturition is depleted or insufficient anticoagulant proteins concentration. Indeed, women with preterm labor without intra-amniotic infection or inflammation and those with vaginal bleeding who delivered preterm had a lower median maternal plasma protein Z, a co-factor that participate in the inhibition of factor Xa, concentration than women with normal pregnancy and those with vaginal bleeding who delivered at term [86]. Moreover, both patients with preterm labor and preterm PROM had a lower median maternal plasma concentration of total tissue factor pathway inhibitor (TFPI), the main physiological inhibitor of the TF pathway, regardless of the presence of infection or gestational age at delivery. These observations suggest that the increased thrombin generation observed among these patients may derive not only from an increased activation of the hemostatic system, but also from insufficient anti-coagulation. The latter can be due to either low concentrations of the anticoagulant proteins, or as a result of an abnormal balance between coagulation factors and their inhibitors.

The overall balance between the concentration and activity of the coagulation factors and the anti-coagulation proteins is one of the determining factors of thrombin generation. In the normal state, the immunoreactive concentrations of TFPI in the plasma are 500 to 1000 times higher than that of TF [87], suggesting that an excess of anti-coagulant proteins closely controls the coagulation cascade activity [87]. Although preterm labor was not associated with a significant change in the median maternal plasma tissue factor concentration, the TFPI/TF ratio was lower than that of normal pregnant women, mainly due to decreased TFPI concentrations. Along with the reports that patients with preterm PROM [72], as well as those with preeclampsia [88], have a lower median maternal plasma TFPI/TF ratio than that of normal pregnant women. The lower TFPI/TF ratio in patients with preeclampsia occurs despite the increase in the median maternal plasma TFPI concentration observed in these patients. This suggests that the balance between TF and its natural inhibitor may better reflect the overall activity of the TF pathway of coagulation, than the individual concentrations of TF or TFPI. Collectively, these observations suggest that our attention should be focused not only on the coagulation protein but also on their inhibitors since an imbalance between them may contribute to increased thrombin generation leading to the activation of preterm parturition.

Inflammation is a major process in term and pre term parturition. In recent years it has become apparent that tight and reciprocal interactions exist between coagulation and inflammation [90]. Originally, much attention was given to mechanisms by which inflammatory mediators, most notably cytokines, can activate coagulation. More recent investigations have revealed that, in turn, mediators involved in the regulation of coagulation and anticoagulation have major effects on the inflammatory processes.

Inflammation elicits coagulation primarily by activating the tissue factor pathway [89] and the generation of thrombin and fibrin. The pivotal role of tissue factor in activation of coagulation during a systemic inflammatory response syndrome, such as produced by endotoxemia or severe sepsis, is well established, and attenuation of the activation of the tissue factor/factor VIIa pathway in endotoxemic humans and chimpanzees and in bacteremic baboons abrogated the activation of the common pathway of coagulation [90-92] and decreased the morbidity associated with these systemic inflammatory conditions.

During preterm PROM and preterm labor, there is a moderate maternal systemic inflammation that results in monocyte and granulocyte activation [75]. Activated monocytes express TF on their membrane [93-97] and shed micro-particles containing TF into the plasma [93]. In addition, the lack of association between intra-amniotic infection/inflammation, as well as the placental histologic findings and median maternal plasma concentrations of TF and TFPI, suggest that the pro-coagulant changes observed in patients with preterm PROM may be due to a systemic rather than a local (i.e. placental, intrauterine) inflammatory process.

Moreover, preterm PROM is associated with an increased activation of the decidual component of the common pathway of parturition [98]. Thus, in pregnancies complicated by abnormal placentation or intrauterine infection, decidual bleeding may lead to a higher expression of TF and activation of the coagulation cascade, resulting in increased thrombin generation. The latter has uterotonic properties that may generate uterine contractions that could initiate labor [70,79,80]. Moreover, thrombin can mediate the activation of MMP-1 [78], MMP-3 [77], and MMP-9[99] that can digest components of the extracellular matrix, weaken the chorioamniotic membranes and predispose to preterm PROM.

The mechanisms described above are localized to the maternal-fetal interface. The lack of association between median maternal plasma TF concentrations and the presence of intra-amniotic infection/inflammation or vaginal bleeding in patients with preterm PROM suggest that the systemic maternal inflammatory response during preterm PROM[75] may contribute the increase median maternal plasma TF concentration in these patients regardless to the presence of infection or inflammation in the amniotic cavity or the occurrence of vaginal bleeding [100].

In addition to the maternal circulation intra-amniotic infection and/or inflammation is associated with an increased amniotic fluid TAT III complexes (figure 7). This is important since it represent an increased thrombin generation in the amniotic cavity during infection and or inflammation that may contribute to uterine contractility and the development of preterm birth [99]. Of interest, elevated intra-amniotic TAT III concentrations were associated with a shorter amniocentesis to delivery interval and an earlier gestational age at delivery only inpatients with preterm labor without intra-amniotic infection or inflammation [99]. This observation suggest that in a subset of patients with preterm labor activation of the coagulation system can generate preterm parturition and delivery; while in those with intra-amniotic infection and or inflammation the activation of the coagulation and thrombin generation is a byproduct of the inflammatory process leading to preterm birth.

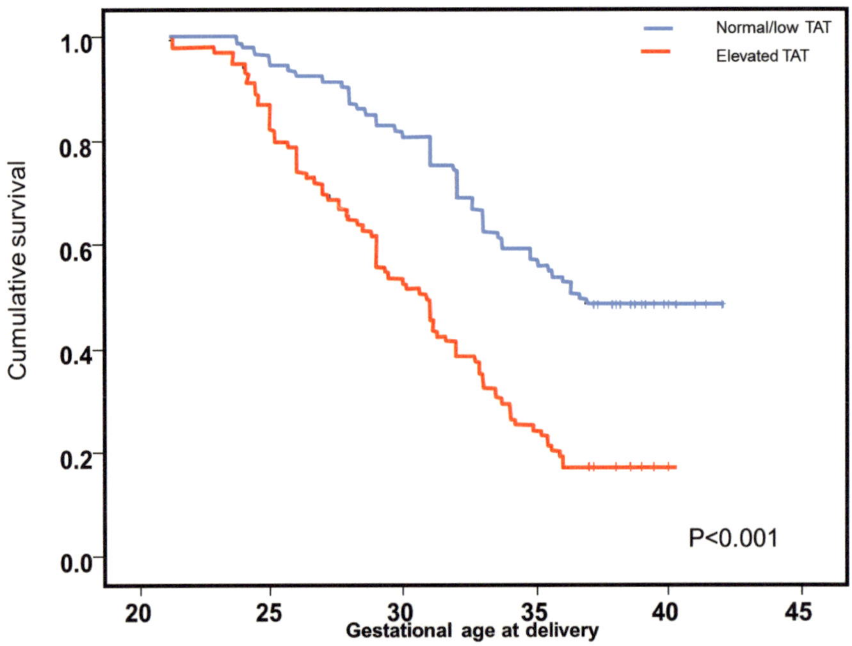

Figure 7. The effect of amniotic fluid thrombin-antithrombin (TAT) III concentrations on gestational age at delivery (from reference #69 with permission)

5. Placental vascular changes in women with preterm parturition

Accumulating evidence from studies of the placenta [101,102], uterine artery Doppler scans [103], and animal experiments [104], suggest a role for uteroplacental ischemia in preterm birth. Indeed, Arias et al reported that about 20% of the placentas of patients who delivered preterm following preterm labor or preterm PROM had vascular lesions [105].

http://dx.doi.org/10.5772/54843

The invasion of trophoblast cells into the decidual and myometrial segments of the spiral arteries is a key point of normal placentation. This process results in reversible changes of the normal spiral arteries wall architecture [106]. The ''disappearance of the normal muscular and elastic structures of the arteries and their replacement by fibrinoid material in which trophoblast cells are embedded'' was originally termed physiologic transformation by Brosens et al in 1967. This process progressively remodeled, starting from the end of the first trimester onward, the uterine spiral arteries to form dilated conduits lacking maternal vasomotor control, ensuring the delivery of a constant supply of blood to the maternal-fetal interface at an optimal velocity for nutrient exchange [107]. Notably, several coagulation components, such as TF and thrombomodulin, are involved not only in hemostasis but also with placental blood vessel differentiation [38,42], affecting thereby the generation of different pathological condition affecting pregnancy and parturition; A higher rate of failure of transformation of the spiral arteries was reported in placentas of patients with preterm labor and preterm PROM than in those of normal pregnant women. This lesion has been implicated in the increased vascular resistance in the placental bed and the reduction of blood flow to the intervillous space [108,109], this is considered as a marker for defective placentation. Failure of transformation of the spiral artery was first reported in women with preeclampsia [110]. Indeed, the extent of this lesion in placenta of women with preeclampsia is more extensive than what is detected in women with preterm labor or preterm PROM [111-113], suggesting when extensive failure of physiologic transformation is present, narrowed uteroplacental arteries predispose to reduced perfusion of the intervillous space, ischemia, and compensatory maternal hypertension. If these lesions are less extensive, the degree of ischemia may be insufficient to induce maternal hypertension, but may predispose to preterm labor/preterm delivery by itself or in association with other pathologic processes, such as intrauterine infection. A report that support the concept that clinical presentation is somewhat reflecting the extent of the disease is the study by Espinoza et al who found that women with an episode of preterm labor who delivered at term had a higher rate of SGA neonates and increased frequency of placental vascular lesions in comparison to those with preterm labor who delivered preterm [114]. This finding suggests that in some cases the vascular lesions that lead to development of preterm labor is not severe enough to cause preterm birth, however the "price" for the continuum of the pregnancy to term is decrease fetal growth.

6. The future — Hemostatic markers for preterm parturition?

In light of the association between maternal plasma TAT III concentrations in women with preterm labor and preterm birth within a week; and the association between amniotic fluid TAT III concentrations, the interval from amniocentesis to delivery, and gestational age at delivery. The question of the role of hemostatic markers as predictors for preterm birth is relevant. A preliminary report by Vidaeff et al found that increased concentrations of amniotic fluid TAT III concentration during mid-trimester amniocentesis of asymptomatic patients is associated with subsequent preterm delivery [115]. Aside the amniotic fluid new assays that study the thrombin generation potential in maternal blood may offer similar answer in less invasive methods [116].

7. Conclusions

The understanding of the homeostasis system and coagulation process is crucial for understanding the physiological and pathological parturition. The significant impact of placentation abnormalities caused by those same changes in the haemostatic system, on maternal and fetal wellbeing is yet to be studied.

The aim of this chapter was to provide a window to the complexity of the normal homeostasis and pregnancy and a view of the different pathological conditions that may emerge during parturition. The inflammation as well as the coagulation and placental implantation are all part of the total picture of parturition.

Author details

Vered Klaitman, Ruth Beer-Wiesel, Tal Rafaeli, Moshe Mazor and Offer Erez

*Address all correspondence to: erezof@bgu.ac.il

Department of Obstetrics and Gynecology "B", Soroka University Medical Center, School of Medicine, Faculty of Health Sciences, Ben Gurion University of the Negev, Beer Sheva, Israel

References

[1] Rand JH, Wu XX, Potter BJ, Uson RR, Gordon RE. Co-localization of von Willebrand factor and type VI collagen in human vascular subendothelium. Am J Pathol 1993 Mar; 142(3):843-850.

[2] Ruggeri ZM, Dent JA, Saldívar E. Contribution of Distinct Adhesive Interactions to Platelet Aggregation in Flowing Blood. Blood 1999 July 01;94(1):172-178.

[3] Nurden AT, Nurden P. A review of the role of platelet membrane glycoproteins in the platelet-vessel wall interaction. Baillieres Clin Haematol 1993 Sep;6(3):653-690.

[4] Pytela R, Pierschbacher MD, Ginsberg MH, Plow EF, Ruoslahti E. Platelet membrane glycoprotein IIb/IIIa: member of a family of Arg-Gly-Asp--specific adhesion receptors. Science 1986 Mar 28;231(4745):1559-1562.

[5] Lockwood CJ. Pregnancy-associated changes in the hemostatic system. Clin Obstet Gynecol 2006 Dec;49(4):836-843.

[6] Greer P., Forster J., Lukens JN., Rodgers GM., Paraskevas F., Glader B. Wintrobs clinical hematology. : Lippincott, Williams and Wilkins; 2004.

[7] Key NS, Geng JG, Bach RR. Tissue factor; from Morawitz to microparticles. Trans Am Clin Climatol Assoc 2007;118:165-173.

[8] Rao LVM, Pendurthi UR. Tissue Factor–Factor VIIa Signaling. Arteriosclerosis, Thrombosis, and Vascular Biology ;25(1):47-56.

[9] Semeraro N, Colucci M. Tissue factor in health and disease. Thromb Haemost 1997 Jul; 78(1):759-764.

[10] Mackman N, Sawdey MS, Keeton MR, Loskutoff DJ. Murine tissue factor gene expression in vivo. Tissue and cell specificity and regulation by lipopolysaccharide. Am J Pathol 1993 Jul;143(1):76-84.

[11] Drake TA, Morrissey JH, Edgington TS. Selective cellular expression of tissue factor in human tissues. Implications for disorders of hemostasis and thrombosis. Am J Pathol 1989 May;134(5):1087-1097.

[12] ADAMS RLC, BIRD RJ. Review article: Coagulation cascade and therapeutics update: Relevance to nephrology. Part 1: Overview of coagulation, thrombophilias and history of anticoagulants. Nephrology 2009;14(5):462-470.

[13] Guller S, Tang Z, Ma YY, Di Santo S, Sager R, Schneider H. Protein composition of microparticles shed from human placenta during placental perfusion: Potential role in angiogenesis and fibrinolysis in preeclampsia. Placenta 2011 Jan;32(1):63-69.

[14] Piccin A, Murphy WG, Smith OP. Circulating microparticles: pathophysiology and clinical implications. Blood Rev 2007 May;21(3):157-171.

[15] Sturk-Maquelin KN, Nieuwland R, Romijn FP, Eijsman L, Hack CE, Sturk A. Pro- and non-coagulant forms of non-cell-bound tissue factor in vivo. J Thromb Haemost 2003 Sep;1(9):1920-1926.

[16] Marlar R, Kleiss A, Griffin J. An alternative extrinsic pathway of human blood coagulation. Blood 1982 December 01;60(6):1353-1358.

[17] Mackman N, Tilley RE, Key NS. Role of the Extrinsic Pathway of Blood Coagulation in Hemostasis and Thrombosis. Arteriosclerosis, Thrombosis, and Vascular Biology 2007 August 01;27(8):1687-1693.

[18] Greenwalt TJ. The how and why of exocytic vesicles. Transfusion 2006;46(1):143-152.

[19] Ranby M, Brandstrom A. Biological control of tissue plasminogen activator-mediated fibrinolysis. Enzyme 1988;40(2-3):130-143.

[20] Schatz F, Lockwood CJ. Progestin regulation of plasminogen activator inhibitor type 1 in primary cultures of endometrial stromal and decidual cells. Journal of Clinical Endocrinology & Metabolism 1993 September 01;77(3):621-625.

[21] Lanir N, Aharon A, Brenner B. Procoagulant and anticoagulant mechanisms in human placenta. Semin Thromb Hemost 2003 Apr;29(2):175-184.

[22] Bouma BN, Meijers JC. New insights into factors affecting clot stability: A role for thrombin activatable fibrinolysis inhibitor (TAFI; plasma procarboxypeptidase B, plasma procarboxypeptidase U, procarboxypeptidase R). Semin Hematol 2004 Jan;41(1 Suppl 1):13-19.

[23] Ku DH, Arkel YS, Paidas MP, Lockwood CJ. Circulating levels of inflammatory cytokines (IL-1 beta and TNF-alpha), resistance to activated protein C, thrombin and fibrin generation in uncomplicated pregnancies. Thromb Haemost 2003 Dec;90(6): 1074-1079.

[24] Urano T, Ihara H, Takada Y, Nagai N, Takada A. The inhibition of human factor Xa by plasminogen activator inhibitor type 1 in the presence of calcium ion, and its enhancement by heparin and vitronectin. Biochim Biophys Acta 1996 Dec 5;1298(2):199-208.

[25] Yuen PM, Yin JA, Lao TT. Fibrinopeptide A levels in maternal and newborn plasma. Eur J Obstet Gynecol Reprod Biol 1989 Mar;30(3):239-244.

[26] Sorensen JD, Secher NJ, Jespersen J. Perturbed (procoagulant) endothelium and deviations within the fibrinolytic system during the third trimester of normal pregnancy. A possible link to placental function. Acta Obstet Gynecol Scand 1995 Apr;74(4): 257-261.

[27] Walker MC, Garner PR, Keely EJ, Rock GA, Reis MD. Changes in activated protein C resistance during normal pregnancy. Am J Obstet Gynecol 1997 Jul;177(1):162-169.

[28] Bellart J, Gilabert R, Miralles RM, Monasterio J, Cabero L. Endothelial cell markers and fibrinopeptide A to D-dimer ratio as a measure of coagulation and fibrinolysis balance in normal pregnancy. Gynecol Obstet Invest 1998;46(1):17-21.

[29] de Boer K, ten Cate JW, Sturk A, Borm JJ, Treffers PE. Enhanced thrombin generation in normal and hypertensive pregnancy. Am J Obstet Gynecol 1989 Jan;160(1):95-100.

[30] Chaiworapongsa T, Espinoza J, Yoshimatsu J, Kim YM, Bujold E, Edwin S, et al. Activation of coagulation system in preterm labor and preterm premature rupture of membranes. J Matern Fetal Neonatal Med 2002 11(6):368-373.

[31] Yoneyama Y, Suzuki S, Sawa R, Otsubo Y, Power GG, Araki T. Plasma adenosine levels increase in women with normal pregnancies. Am J Obstet Gynecol 2000 May;182(5): 1200-1203.

[32] Sheu JR, Hsiao G, Luk HN, Chen YW, Chen TL, Lee LW, et al. Mechanisms involved in the antiplatelet activity of midazolam in human platelets. Anesthesiology 2002 Mar; 96(3):651-658.

[33] Bremme KA. Haemostatic changes in pregnancy. Best Pract Res Clin Haematol 2003 Jun;16(2):153-168.

[34] Eichinger S, Weltermann A, Philipp K, Hafner E, Kaider A, Kittl EM, et al. Prospective evaluation of hemostatic system activation and thrombin potential in healthy pregnant women with and without factor V Leiden. Thromb Haemost 1999 Oct;82(4):1232-1236.

[35] Faught W, Garner P, Jones G, Ivey B. Changes in protein C and protein S levels in normal pregnancy. Am J Obstet Gynecol 1995 Jan;172(1 Pt 1):147-150.

[36] Craven CM, Chedwick LR, Ward K. Placental basal plate formation is associated with fibrin deposition in decidual veins at sites of trophoblast cell invasion. Am J Obstet Gynecol 2002 Feb;186(2):291-296.

[37] Sheppard BL, Bonnar J. Uteroplacental hemostasis in intrauterine fetal growth retardation. Semin Thromb Hemost 1999;25(5):443-446.

[38] Lockwood CJ, Krikun G, Runic R, Schwartz LB, Mesia AF, Schatz F. Progestin-epidermal growth factor regulation of tissue factor expression during decidualization of human endometrial stromal cells. J Clin Endocrinol Metab 2000 Jan;85(1):297-301.

[39] Beller FK, Ebert C. The coagulation and fibrinolytic enzyme system in pregnancy and in the puerperium. Eur J Obstet Gynecol Reprod Biol 1982 May;13(3):177-197.

[40] Schatz F, Krikun G, Caze R, Rahman M, Lockwood CJ. Progestin-regulated expression of tissue factor in decidual cells: implications in endometrial hemostasis, menstruation and angiogenesis. Steroids 2003 Nov;68(10-13):849-860.

[41] Clark P, Brennand J, Conkie JA, McCall F, Greer IA, Walker ID. Activated protein C sensitivity, protein C, protein S and coagulation in normal pregnancy. Thromb Haemost 1998 Jun;79(6):1166-1170.

[42] Brenner B. Haemostatic changes in pregnancy. Thromb Res 2004;114(5–6):409-414.

[43] Udagawa K, Miyagi Y, Hirahara F, Miyagi E, Nagashima Y, Minaguchi H, et al. Specific expression of PP5/TFPI2 mRNA by syncytiotrophoblasts in human placenta as revealed by in situ hybridization. Placenta 1998 Mar-Apr;19(2-3):217-223.

[44] Udagawa K, Yasumitsu H, Esaki M, Sawada H, Nagashima Y, Aoki I, et al. Subcellular localization of PP5/TFPI-2 in human placenta: a possible role of PP5/TFPI-2 as an anti-coagulant on the surface of syncytiotrophoblasts. Placenta 2002 Feb-Mar;23(2-3): 145-153.

[45] Salem HT, Menabawey M, Seppala M, Shaaban MM, Chard T. Human seminal plasma contains a wide range of trophoblast-'specific' proteins. Placenta 1984 Sep-Oct;5(5): 413-417.

[46] Salem HT, Chard T. Placental protein 5 (PP5): biological and clinical studies. Placenta Suppl 1982;4:103-114.

[47] Lee JN, Salem HT, Chard T, Huang SC, Ouyang PC. Circulating placental proteins (hCG, SP1 and PP5) in trophoblastic disease. Br J Obstet Gynaecol 1982 Jan;89(1):69-72.

[48] Rohde LH, Carson DD. Heparin-like glycosaminoglycans participate in binding of a human trophoblastic cell line (JAR) to a human uterine epithelial cell line (RL95). J Cell Physiol 1993 Apr;155(1):185-196.

[49] Gonzalez M, Neufeld J, Reimann K, Wittmann S, Samalecos A, Wolf A, et al. Expansion of human trophoblastic spheroids is promoted by decidualized endometrial stromal cells and enhanced by heparin-binding epidermal growth factor-like growth factor and interleukin-1 beta. Mol Hum Reprod 2011 Jul;17(7):421-433.

[50] Maruyama I, Bell CE, Majerus PW. Thrombomodulin is found on endothelium of arteries, veins, capillaries, and lymphatics, and on syncytiotrophoblast of human placenta. J Cell Biol 1985 Aug;101(2):363-371.

[51] Leach L, Bhasin Y, Clark P, Firth JA. Isolation of endothelial cells from human term placental villi using immunomagnetic beads. Placenta 1994 Jun;15(4):355-364.

[52] Fazel A, Vincenot A, Malassine A, Soncin F, Gaussem P, Alsat E, et al. Increase in expression and activity of thrombomodulin in term human syncytiotrophoblast microvilli. Placenta 1998 May;19(4):261-268.

[53] Sood R, Weiler H. Embryogenesis and gene targeting of coagulation factors in mice. Best Pract Res Clin Haematol 2003 Jun;16(2):169-181.

[54] Reverdiau P, Jarousseau AC, Thibault G, Khalfoun B, Watier H, Lebranchu Y, et al. Tissue factor activity of syncytiotrophoblast plasma membranes and tumoral trophoblast cells in culture. Thromb Haemost 1995 Jan;73(1):49-54.

[55] Crawley JT, Gu JM, Ferrell G, Esmon CT. Distribution of endothelial cell protein C/activated protein C receptor (EPCR) during mouse embryo development. Thromb Haemost 2002 Aug;88(2):259-266.

[56] Hassan SS, Romero R, Tarca AL, Draghici S, Pineles B, Bugrim A, et al. Signature pathways identified from gene expression profiles in the human uterine cervix before and after spontaneous term parturition. Am J Obstet Gynecol 2007 Sep;197(3): 250.e1-250.e7.

[57] Tsatas D, Baker MS, Rice GE. Differential expression of proteases in human gestational tissues before, during and after spontaneous-onset labour at term. J Reprod Fertil 1999 May;116(1):43-49.

[58] Yu Y, Tsai HJ, Liu X, Mestan K, Zhang S, Pearson C, et al. The joint association between F5 gene polymorphisms and maternal smoking during pregnancy on preterm delivery. Hum Genet 2009 Jan;124(6):659-668.

[59] Velez DR, Fortunato SJ, Thorsen P, Lombardi SJ, Williams SM, Menon R. Preterm birth in Caucasians is associated with coagulation and inflammation pathway gene variants. PLoS One 2008 Sep 26;3(9):e3283.

[60] Schjetlein R, Abdelnoor M, Haugen G, Husby H, Sandset PM, Wisloff F. Hemostatic variables as independent predictors for fetal growth retardation in preeclampsia. Acta Obstet Gynecol Scand 1999 Mar;78(3):191-197.

[61] Chaiworapongsa T, Yoshimatsu J, Espinoza J, Kim YM, Berman S, Edwin S, et al. Evidence of in vivo generation of thrombin in patients with small-for-gestational-age fetuses and pre-eclampsia. J Matern Fetal Neonatal Med 2002 Jun;11(6):362-367.

[62] Hayashi M, Numaguchi M, Ohkubo N, Yaoi Y. Blood macrophage colony-stimulating factor and thrombin-antithrombin III complex concentrations in pregnancy and preeclampsia. Am J Med Sci 1998 Apr;315(4):251-257.

[63] Kobayashi T, Terao T. Preeclampsia as chronic disseminated intravascular coagulation. Study of two parameters: thrombin-antithrombin III complex and D-dimers. Gynecol Obstet Invest 1987;24(3):170-178.

[64] Kobayashi T, Tokunaga N, Sugimura M, Suzuki K, Kanayama N, Nishiguchi T, et al. Coagulation/fibrinolysis disorder in patients with severe preeclampsia. Semin Thromb Hemost 1999;25(5):451-454.

[65] Kobayashi T, Sumimoto K, Tokunaga N, Sugimura M, Nishiguchi T, Kanayama N, et al. Coagulation index to distinguish severe preeclampsia from normal pregnancy. Semin Thromb Hemost 2002 Dec;28(6):495-500.

[66] Hayashi M, Inoue T, Hoshimoto K, Negishi H, Ohkura T, Inaba N. Characterization of five marker levels of the hemostatic system and endothelial status in normotensive pregnancy and pre-eclampsia. Eur J Haematol 2002 Nov-Dec;69(5-6):297-302.

[67] Hayashi M, Ohkura T. Elevated levels of serum macrophage colony-stimulating factor in normotensive pregnancies complicated by intrauterine fetal growth restriction. Exp Hematol 2002 May;30(5):388-393.

[68] Ballard HS, Marcus AJ. Primary and secondary platelet aggregation in uraemia. Scand J Haematol 1972;9(3):198-203.

[69] Erez O, Romer R, Vaisbuch E, Chaiworapongsa T, Kusanovic JP, Mazaki-Tovi S, et al. Changes in amniotic fluid concentration of thrombin–antithrombin III complexes in patients with preterm labor: Evidence of an increased thrombin generation. J Matern Fetal Neonatal Med 2009 22(11):971-982.

[70] Elovitz MA, Baron J, Phillippe M. The role of thrombin in preterm parturition. Am J Obstet Gynecol 2001 Nov;185(5):1059-1063.

[71] Rosen T, Kuczynski E, O'Neill LM, Funai EF, Lockwood CJ. Plasma levels of thrombin-antithrombin complexes predict preterm premature rupture of the fetal membranes. J Matern Fetal Med 2001 Oct;10(5):297-300.

[72] Erez O, Espinoza J, Chaiworapongsa T, Gotsch F, Kusanovic JP, Than NG, et al. A link between a hemostatic disorder and preterm PROM: a role for tissue factor and tissue factor pathway inhibitor. J Matern Fetal Neonatal Med 2008 21(10):732-744.

[73] Lockwood CJ, Toti P, Arcuri F, Paidas M, Buchwalder L, Krikun G, et al. Mechanisms of abruption-induced premature rupture of the fetal membranes: thrombin-enhanced interleukin-8 expression in term decidua. Am J Pathol 2005 Nov;167(5):1443-1449.

[74] Gomez R, Romero R, Nien JK, Medina L, Carstens M, Kim YM, et al. Idiopathic vaginal bleeding during pregnancy as the only clinical manifestation of intrauterine infection. J Matern Fetal Neonatal Med 2005 Jul;18(1):31-37.

[75] Gervasi MT, Chaiworapongsa T, Naccasha N, Pacora P, Berman S, Maymon E, et al. Maternal intravascular inflammation in preterm premature rupture of membranes. J Matern Fetal Neonatal Med 2002 Mar;11(3):171-175.

[76] Osterud B, Bjorklid E. Sources of tissue factor. Semin Thromb Hemost 2006 Feb;32(1): 11-23.

[77] Mackenzie AP, Schatz F, Krikun G, Funai EF, Kadner S, Lockwood CJ. Mechanisms of abruption-induced premature rupture of the fetal membranes: Thrombin enhanced decidual matrix metalloproteinase-3 (stromelysin-1) expression. Am J Obstet Gynecol 2004 Dec;191(6):1996-2001.

[78] Rosen T, Schatz F, Kuczynski E, Lam H, Koo AB, Lockwood CJ. Thrombin-enhanced matrix metalloproteinase-1 expression: a mechanism linking placental abruption with premature rupture of the membranes. J Matern Fetal Neonatal Med 2002 Jan;11(1): 11-17.

[79] Elovitz MA, Ascher-Landsberg J, Saunders T, Phillippe M. The mechanisms underlying the stimulatory effects of thrombin on myometrial smooth muscle. Am J Obstet Gynecol 2000 Sep;183(3):674-681.

[80] Elovitz MA, Saunders T, Ascher-Landsberg J, Phillippe M. Effects of thrombin on myometrial contractions in vitro and in vivo. Am J Obstet Gynecol 2000 Oct;183(4): 799-804.

[81] Lockwood CJ, Krikun G, Schatz F. Decidual cell-expressed tissue factor maintains hemostasis in human endometrium. Ann N Y Acad Sci 2001 Sep;943:77-88.

[82] Lockwood CJ, Krikun G, Schatz F. The decidua regulates hemostasis in human endometrium. Semin Reprod Endocrinol 1999;17(1):45-51.

[83] Lockwood CJ, Schatz F. A biological model for the regulation of peri-implantational hemostasis and menstruation. J Soc Gynecol Investig 1996 Jul-Aug;3(4):159-165.

[84] Hahn L. On fibrinolysis and coagulation during parturition and menstruation. Acta Obstet Gynecol Scand Suppl 1974;28:7-40.

[85] Major CA, de Veciana M, Lewis DF, Morgan MA. Preterm premature rupture of membranes and abruptio placentae: is there an association between these pregnancy complications? Am J Obstet Gynecol 1995 Feb;172(2 Pt 1):672-676.

[86] Kusanovic JP, Espinoza J, Romero R, Hoppensteadt D, Nien JK, Kim CJ, et al. Plasma protein Z concentrations in pregnant women with idiopathic intrauterine bleeding and

in women with spontaneous preterm labor. J Matern Fetal Neonatal Med 2007 Jun;20(6): 453-463.

[87] Shimura M, Wada H, Wakita Y, Nakase T, Hiyoyama K, Nagaya S, et al. Plasma tissue factor and tissue factor pathway inhibitor levels in patients with disseminated intravascular coagulation. Am J Hematol 1997 Aug;55(4):169-174.

[88] Erez O, Romero R, Hoppensteadt D, Than NG, Fareed J, Mazaki-Tovi S, et al. Tissue factor and its natural inhibitor in pre-eclampsia and SGA. J Matern Fetal Neonatal Med 2008 Dec;21(12):855-869.

[89] Levi M, van der Poll T. Inflammation and coagulation. Crit Care Med 2010 Feb;38(2 Suppl):S26-34.

[90] van der Poll T, Levi M, Hack CE, ten Cate H, van Deventer SJ, Eerenberg AJ, et al. Elimination of interleukin 6 attenuates coagulation activation in experimental endotoxemia in chimpanzees. J Exp Med 1994 Apr 1;179(4):1253-1259.

[91] van der Poll T, de Boer JD, Levi M. The effect of inflammation on coagulation and vice versa. Curr Opin Infect Dis 2011 Jun;24(3):273-278.

[92] Schouten M, Wiersinga WJ, Levi M, van der Poll T. Inflammation, endothelium, and coagulation in sepsis. J Leukoc Biol 2008 Mar;83(3):536-545.

[93] Butenas S, Bouchard BA, Brummel-Ziedins KE, Parhami-Seren B, Mann KG. Tissue factor activity in whole blood. Blood 2005 Apr 1;105(7):2764-2770.

[94] Osterud B. Cellular interactions in tissue factor expression by blood monocytes. Blood Coagul Fibrinolysis 1995 Jun;6 Suppl 1:S20-5.

[95] Rivers RP, Hathaway WE, Weston WL. The endotoxin-induced coagulant activity of human monocytes. Br J Haematol 1975 Jul;30(3):311-316.

[96] Bach RR, Moldow CF. Mechanism of tissue factor activation on HL-60 cells. Blood 1997 May 1;89(9):3270-3276.

[97] Egorina EM, Sovershaev MA, Bjorkoy G, Gruber FX, Olsen JO, Parhami-Seren B, et al. Intracellular and surface distribution of monocyte tissue factor: application to intersubject variability. Arterioscler Thromb Vasc Biol 2005 Jul;25(7):1493-1498.

[98] Romero R, Espinoza J, Kusanovic JP, Gotsch F, Hassan S, Erez O, et al. The preterm parturition syndrome. BJOG 2006 Dec;113 Suppl 3:17-42.

[99] Stephenson CD, Lockwood CJ, Ma Y, Guller S. Thrombin-dependent regulation of matrix metalloproteinase (MMP)-9 levels in human fetal membranes. J Matern Fetal Neonatal Med 2005 Jul;18(1):17-22.

[100] Erez O, Romero R, Vaisbuch E, Kusanovic JP, Mazaki-Tovi S, Chaiworapongsa T, et al. High tissue factor activity and low tissue factor pathway inhibitor concentrations in patients with preterm labor. J Matern Fetal Neonatal Med 2010 23(1):23-33.

[101] Germain AM, Carvajal J, Sanchez M, Valenzuela GJ, Tsunekawa H, Chuaqui B. Preterm labor: placental pathology and clinical correlation. Obstet Gynecol 1999 Aug;94(2): 284-289.

[102] Arias F, Rodriquez L, Rayne SC, Kraus FT. Maternal placental vasculopathy and infection: two distinct subgroups among patients with preterm labor and preterm ruptured membranes. Am J Obstet Gynecol 1993 Feb;168(2):585-591.

[103] Strigini FA, Lencioni G, De Luca G, Lombardo M, Bianchi F, Genazzani AR. Uterine artery velocimetry and spontaneous preterm delivery. Obstet Gynecol 1995 Mar;85(3): 374-377.

[104] Combs CA, Katz MA, Kitzmiller JL, Brescia RJ. Experimental preeclampsia produced by chronic constriction of the lower aorta: validation with longitudinal blood pressure measurements in conscious rhesus monkeys. Am J Obstet Gynecol 1993 Jul;169(1): 215-223.

[105] Arias F, Victoria A, Cho K, Kraus F. Placental histology and clinical characteristics of patients with preterm premature rupture of membranes. Obstet Gynecol 1997 Feb; 89(2):265-271.

[106] Pijnenborg R, Bland JM, Robertson WB, Brosens I. Uteroplacental arterial changes related to interstitial trophoblast migration in early human pregnancy. Placenta 1983 Oct-Dec;4(4):397-413.

[107] Brosens I, Robertson WB, Dixon HG. The physiological response of the vessels of the placental bed to normal pregnancy. J Pathol Bacteriol 1967 Apr;93(2):569-579.

[108] Kim YM, Bujold E, Chaiworapongsa T, Gomez R, Yoon BH, Thaler HT, et al. Failure of physiologic transformation of the spiral arteries in patients with preterm labor and intact membranes. Am J Obstet Gynecol 2003 Oct;189(4):1063-1069.

[109] Kim YM, Chaiworapongsa T, Gomez R, Bujold E, Yoon BH, Rotmensch S, et al. Failure of physiologic transformation of the spiral arteries in the placental bed in preterm premature rupture of membranes. Am J Obstet Gynecol 2002 Nov;187(5):1137-1142.

[110] Brosens IA, Robertson WB, Dixon HG. The role of the spiral arteries in the pathogenesis of preeclampsia. Obstet Gynecol Annu 1972;1:177-191.

[111] Khong Y, Brosens I. Defective deep placentation. Best Pract Res Clin Obstet Gynaecol 2011 Jun;25(3):301-311.

[112] Espinoza J, Romero R, Mee Kim Y, Kusanovic JP, Hassan S, Erez O, et al. Normal and abnormal transformation of the spiral arteries during pregnancy. J Perinat Med 2006;34(6):447-458.

[113] Brosens I, Pijnenborg R, Vercruysse L, Romero R. The "Great Obstetrical Syndromes" are associated with disorders of deep placentation. Am J Obstet Gynecol 2011 Mar; 204(3):193-201.

[114] Espinoza J, Kusanovic JP, Kim CJ, Kim YM, Kim JS, Hassan SS, et al. An episode of preterm labor is a risk factor for the birth of a small-for-gestational-age neonate. Am J Obstet Gynecol 2007 Jun;196(6):574.e1-5; discussion 574.e5-6.

[115] Vidaeff AC, Monga M, Saade G, Bishop K, Ramin SM. Prospective investigation of second-trimester thrombin activation and preterm birth. Am J Obstet Gynecol 2012 Apr;206(4):333.e1-333.e6.

[116] Hackney DN, Catov JM, Simhan HN. Low concentrations of thrombin-inhibitor complexes and the risk of preterm delivery. Am J Obstet Gynecol 2010 Aug;203(2): 184.e1-184.e6.

Chapter 4

Placenta in Preterm Birth

Erdener Ozer

Additional information is available at the end of the chapter

http://dx.doi.org/10.5772/54887

1. Introduction

This chapter provides an understanding of specific patterns of placental pathology and their associations with the various phenotypes and underlying mechanisms of preterm birth.

To the perinatal pathologists, preterm births are those occurring at less than 37 weeks of gestation. In almost all countries with reliable data, preterm birth rates have increased worldwide. The complications of preterm birth due to prematurity are often serious community health problems and account for 75% of perinatal mortalities and more than 50% of long-term infant morbidities [1]. Globally, prematurity is the leading cause of newborn deaths and now the second leading cause of death after pneumonia in children under the age of five [2]. The complications of prematurity include adverse cognitive, organ functional and motor outcomes. Moreover, preterm infants have increased rates chronic lung disease, necrotizing enterocolitis and neurological sequels including periventricular leukomalacia. Later in childhood, they have reduced motor, intellectual and behavioral skills compared to children born at term.

Clinical managements to reduce the incidence of preterm birth have not been yet very successful. They have largely been targeting treatments for individual risk factors and focused on answering clinical questions rather than pathogenic mechanisms such as placental ones. The above facts regarding the clinical importance of preterm birth reveal that the pathologist is and will be increasingly asked to examine placentas from preterm births in order to help explaining the pathogenesis of preterm birth. In addition, the placental examinations from these cases may provide valuable clues for predicting which infants and *why* some infants may be at relatively greater risk for developing long term complications of preterm births.

The aim of this chapter is to present sufficient pathogenic background concerning what is currently appreciated about the placental pathology in preterm birth in order that the practicing perinatologists will be aware of the fact that any infant requiring the care of a neonatologist should have a placental examination.

2. Clinicopathological scenarios

The causes of singleton preterm birth are incompletely understood, and a full discussion of the current clinical literature on this subject is beyond the scope of this chapter. Supporting the fetus through the preceding gestation, the placenta is a very critical organ in explaining the pathogenesis of preterm birth. From this point of view, the placental pathology will be emphasized in two clinical categories of preterm birth: spontaneous preterm birth (SPB) and indicated preterm birth (IPB).

SPB can be classified into two separate clinical scenarios: (i) premature onset of labor (POL) defined as regular contractions with accompanying cervical change and with intact membranes, and accounting for 40–45% of cases of preterm births or (ii) preterm premature rupture of membranes (PPROM) defined as spontaneous rupture of membranes at less than 37 weeks of gestation and at least one hour before the onset of contractions, and seen in 25–30% of preterm births) [1].

IPB is defined when the labor is induced or caesarean section is performed for maternal or fetal reasons. It has a high frequency of associated maternal vascular changes in the placenta, similar to those described for hypertension or diabetes, as well as placental abruptions.

3. Placental pathology in spontaneous preterm birth

The various pathologic reaction patterns in SPB can be grouped in etiological context by determining whether the etiological process is infectious or non-microbial (Table 1). There is a large body of evidence that a cascade of activations of cellular components and mediators of inflammatory pathways result in onset of labor and membrane rupture [3, 4]. POL and PPROM are likely to be the pathological results of abnormal microbial and non-microbial activation of imbalances among these normally orchestrated components and mediators.

POL may result from (i) acute chorioamnionitis, (ii) uteroplacental underperfusion, (iii) uterine fundal and cervical abnormalities or fetal anomalies. However, non-microbial etiologies appear more prevalent. Acute uteroplacental underperfusion may be due to a retroplacental hemorrhage (placental abruption). Chronic uteroplacental underperfusion is seen in maternal chronic hypertension or diabetes.

The placenta in PPROM often shows evidence of ascending infection (amniotic fluid infection sequence) or vasculopathic problems (hemorrhage or thrombi). Amniotic fluid infection has clinical significance for the neonate beyond just causing preterm birth. The fetus may reveal an inflammatory response associated with cytokine release that can cause damage to the

Infectious etiology	Acute inflammatory pathology	1. Acute chorioamnionitis
		- *Subacute chorioamnionitis*
		2. Acute villitis
	Chronic inflammatory pathology	1. Chronic villitis
		- *CMV placentitis*
		- *Syphilis placentitis*
		- *HSV placentitis*
		2. Idiopathic chronic deciduitis
Non-microbial etiology	1. Retromembranous hemorrhage	
	2. Retroplacental hematoma	
	3. Marginal hematoma	
	4. Uteroplacental underperfusion	

Table 1. Etiopathogenetic correlation of placental pathology in spontaneous preterm birth

developing brain and lungs. This inflammatory response is evident microscopically by neutrophils migrating from the fetal vasculature of the umbilical cord or chorionic plate towards the infected amnionic fluid.

4. Placental pathology of intrauterine infections and inflammatory processes in SPB

Intrauterine infection is clinically a common etiology of SPB following POL and PPROM. It is most prevalent and severe in early preterm infant. Bacterial infection is very common and predisposes to preterm delivery. The most common pathogens include the genital mycoplasmas (especially *Ureaplasma urealyticum*) and *Streptococcus agalactiae, Escherichia coli, Fusobacterium,* and *Gardnerella vaginalis* [4]. Group B streptococcus, *Staphylococcus, Propionibacterium, Peptostreptococcus, Pseudomonas, Proteus* and *Klebsiella* species have also been commonly detected [5]. Although *Candida albicans* is an uncommon pathogen, it has been associated with high rates of morbidity and mortality in earlier cases of preterm birth.

Microbiological studies of amniotic fluid have shown that overall rates of infection in SPB are 25–40%. Approximately 32.5% of women with POL and over 75% with PPROM have positive amniotic fluid cultures. Studies have additionally shown that infection can be confined to the decidua and the rate of chorioamnion colonization is twice that of the amniotic fluid [1]. Although bacterial infection is very common and predisposes to preterm delivery, not all women with positive evidence of bacteria in the chorioamnion have POL or PPROM. In addition, up to 70% of women undergoing elective caesarean section at term have evidence of bacterial invasion and even inflammation [6].

The relative numbers and pathogenicity of the organisms gaining access to the uterine or amniotic fluid cavities, together with the degree of underlying maternal inflammatory response and predisposing genetic, cervical/structural risk factors and/or fetal factors may trigger inflammatory mechanisms involved in normal parturition towards SPB. Based on the observation that 10–15% of placentas at term have histological acute chorioamnionitis, some investigators suggest that chorioamnionitis may develop as a consequence of POL rather than representing a cause of preterm birth [7].

There is a poor correlation between clinically diagnosed chorioamnionitis and the pathological diagnosis of histological acute chorioamnionitis. It can be partly explained by the fact that the clinical definition of chorioamnionitis is non-uniform, and that most cases of histopathological chorioamnionitis represent subclinical infection. Further studies focused on the pathogenetic mechanisms involved in SPB may yield clinicopathological explanations and improved correlations [8].

4.1. Acute chorioamnionitis

Gross examination of the placenta the evidence of chorioamnionitis reveals membranous edema, clouding, or yellowish-green discoloration and congestive placentomegaly. The cord may show punctate yellowish lesions characteristic of candidiasis, although minute whitish lesions may rarely be seen in severe bacterial infections.

The inflammatory response to ascending infection consists of an acute inflammatory neutrophilic infiltrate composed of maternal neutrophils from the intervillous circulation and small venules in the membranous decidua. In many cases this maternal response is supplemented by a fetal response composed of neutrophils emanating from large vessels of the umbilical cord and chorionic plate. Therefore, acute chorioamnionitis should be separated into two components, the maternal and fetal inflammatory responses. Each of these in turn should be characterized in terms of its spatiotemporal progression (stage) and severity (grade) [9].

Maternal inflammatory response begins in the decidua of the external membranes as patchy deciduitis and progresses to margination of neutrophils along the deciduochorionic junction, and additionally infiltration of the subchorionic maternal space. Therefore, the stages of maternal response are;

Stage 1 (early chorioamnionitis or acute subchorionitis): Neutrophils are restricted to subchorionic fibrin and the membranous decidual-chorionic interface.

Stage 2 (acute chorioamnionitis): Neutrophils are located at in chorion and amnion.

Stage 3 (necrotizing chorioamnionitis): There are signs of amnion necrosis including karyorhexis of neutrophils, desquamation of amnionic epithelial cells, and bandlike eosinophilia of the amnionic basement membrane (Figure 1).

Severe maternal inflammatory response responses are characterized by large accumulations of neutrophils (microabcesses) under the chorion. Stage 1 response is generally clinically silent. Stages 2 and 3 are associated with increased risk of neonatal morbidity and mortality. Stage 2 is most common in preterm births, but especially in the earliest periods of gestation [10].

http://dx.doi.org/10.5772/54887

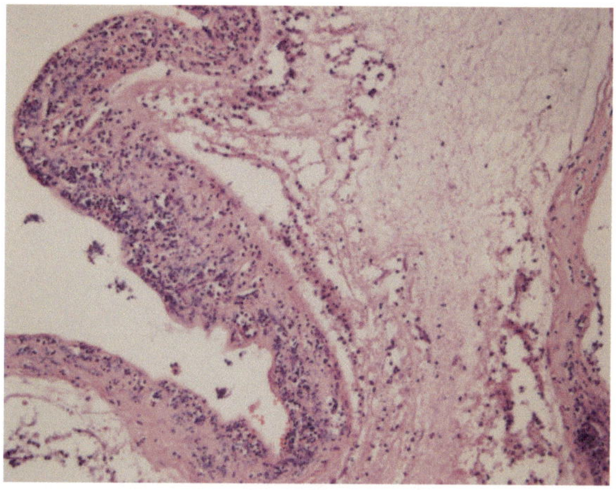

Figure 1. Stage 3 (advanced, late) histological acute chorioamnionitis.

Maternal grade (intensity and distribution of inflammation) 2 of subchorionic neutrophilic aggregation is associated with increased risk of neonatal infection [11].

The fetal inflammatory response to infection is manifested by migration of neutrophils from chorionic plate vessels and from the umbilical cord vessels. Severe fetal responses are characterized by near confluent neutrophilic infiltrates in the amnionic side of chorionic vessels with attenuation and degenerative changes of the vessel wall (Figure 2). The staging of fetal response is;

Stage 1: Neutrophils are located at in chorionic vessels (chorionic vasculitis) and/or umbilical vein (umbilical phlebitis).

Stage 2: There is umbilical arterial infiltration of neutrophils (umbilical arteritis) or trivasculitis (Figure 3).

Stage 3: There are neutrophils and neutrophilic debris forming arcs around umbilical vessels in the Wharton's jelly (necrotizing funisitis).

There are numerous important pathological outcomes associated with fetal inflammatory response stages 2 and 3, and fetal grade 2 (severe), particularly for extremely preterm infants. Fetal grade 2 inflammatory response is characterized by severe inflammation of the cord or chorionic plate vessels and may be accompanied by acute mural non-occlusive thrombosis. Severe fetal response associated with prolonged intrauterine infection may be manifested by necrotizing funisitis revealing mineralization of the inflammatory and debris laden arcs. Fetal stages 2 and 3 generally indicate increasing duration and/or severity of the infection. Fetal grade 2, in particular, is strongly correlated with the presence of high fetal levels of circulating proinflammatory cytokines and inflammatory mediators, such as interleukin-6. This condition is referred to as the fetal inflammatory response syndrome (FIRS). It is currently believed that various aspects of this response including circulating cytokines, bacterial toxins, and activation of the coagulation cascade predispose to cerebral palsy and other forms of adverse neurological

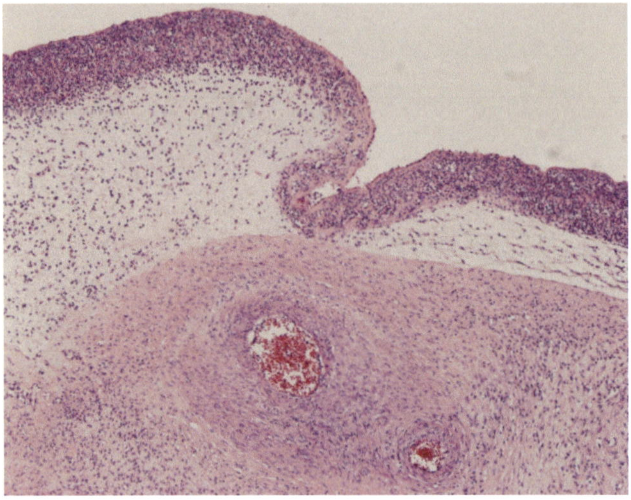

Figure 2. Severe fetal inflammatory response characterized by intense chorionic vasculitis.

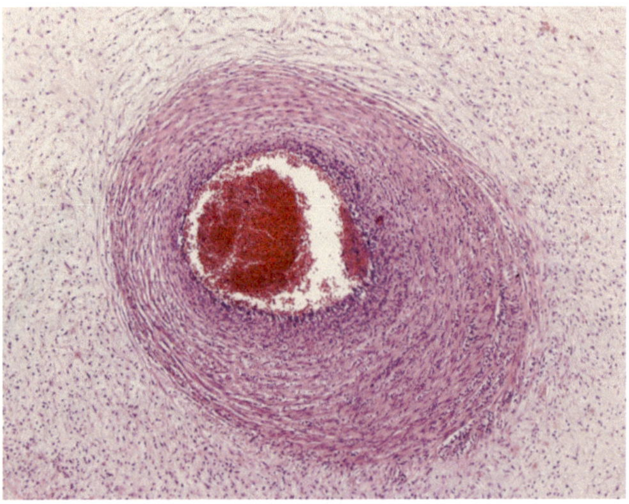

Figure 3. The fetal inflammatory response (stage 2) characterized by funisitis with arteritis.

outcomes, such as periventricular leukomalacia and cerebral palsy. A role for fetal inflammatory response syndrome in the development of chronic lung disease has also been proposed with conflicting evidence.

Chorionic villous edema may also be prominent with fetal grade 2 histopathology. In addition, it has been linked to increased risk in extremely preterm infants, even without intense chorionic vasculitis. The risk is evidenced for cerebral palsy and impaired neurological function when these children reach school age [12]. Thus chorionic villous edemas are potentially an independent histopathological feature associated with increased risk for morbidity and mortality in preterm infants.

Certain organisms have been more strongly associated with both intense chorionic plate inflammation and fetal vasculitis including *Actinomyces* species, *Corynebacterium* species, *Mycoplasma* species, *Escherichia coli*, *Ureaplasma urealyticum* and group B, group D, alpha-hemolytic, and anaerobic streptococci. However, it should be remembered that group B streptococcal infection is not consistently accompanied by significant inflammation. Spread of organisms from the infected placenta to the fetus (so-called early onset sepsis) is rare and chorioamnionitis is rarely a direct cause of intrauterine fetal death. One exception is untreated group B streptococcal infection.

Subacute necrotizing funisitis is a subset of acute chorioamnionitis characterized by peripheral microabscesses of the umbilical cord. The classic gross finding is the presence of pinpoint yellow-white nodules on the umbilical cord that track the coils of the underlying vessels. They are best viewed with tangential light and/or use of a hand-held magnifying lens. These foci correspond to histological subamniotic microabscesses and include mineralization of the arcs of inflammatory detritus. Subacute necrotizing funisitis may also be seen in infections of longer duration and cord vessel thrombosis in more chronic cases. The vast majority of these cases are due to *Candida albicans* but *C parasilopsis* and other species have been identified. Co-infection with bacteria and genital mycoplasmas may also occur.

Intrauterine infection by *Candida*, although a less common cause of acute chorioamnionitis is more prevalent in preterm deliveries and is associated with significant mortality rates in the extreme and severely preterm infant [13]. Gross detection of these lesions at the macroscopy room should need rapid alarming of the neonatologist in charge so that the administration of antifungal therapy can be started, if necessary. In addition, special fungal stains of the lesions should be done. Rarely, the cord lesions represent foci of infections of *Corynebacterium*, *Haemophilus* or *Listeria monocytogenes*.

Subacute chorioamnionitis is another acute inflammatory placental pathology of infectious etiology in SPB. This is a histopathological diagnosis characterized by a chorionic mononuclear (histiocytic) infiltrate admixed with degenerating neutrophils and karyorrhectic debris that is most prominent in the upper zone of the chorionic plate and indicates a more prolonged duration of intrauterine infection. It may represent infection by organisms of low pathogenicity or recurrent mild infection. Clinically it is seen in gestations complicated by repeated second and/or third trimester episodes of bleeding [11].

In a study, it was concluded that subacute chorioamnionitis was strongly associated with the development of chronic lung disease of infancy and that very low birth weight and amniotic necrosis were the strongest predictors of this pulmonary outcome [14]. However, the relative significance of this histopathology needs further investigation. The differential diagnosis includes *chronic, predominantly lymphocytic, chorionitis* which is generally focal and associated with villitis of unknown etiology (Figure 4, 5).

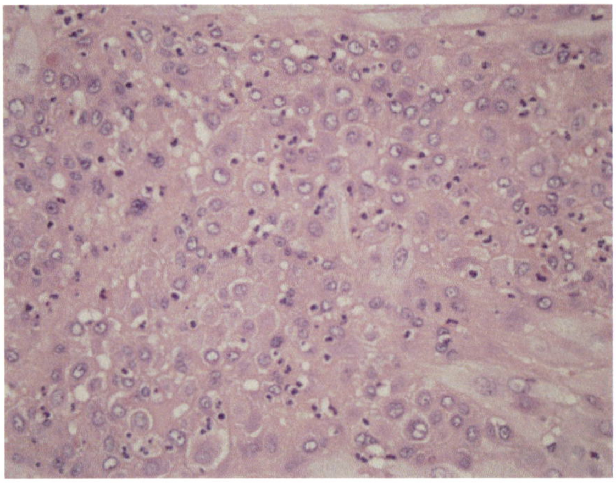

Figure 4. Predominantly lymphocytic focal infiltrate of chronic chorionitis.

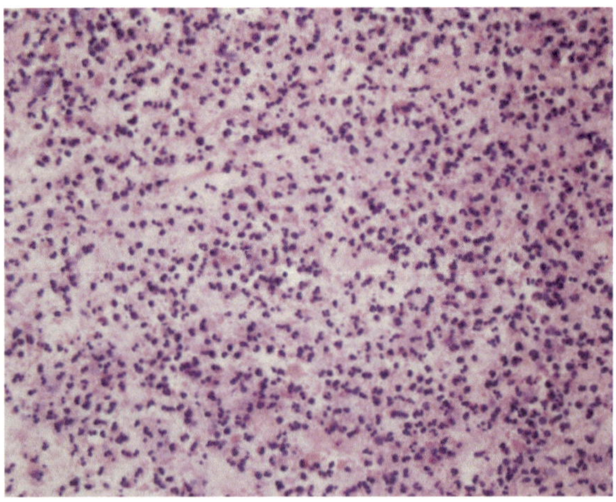

Figure 5. Acute chorionitis characterized by diffuse neutrophilic infiltration

4.2. Acute villitis / intervillositis

This acute inflammatory response is characteristic of hematogenous (transplacental) spread of infection from the mother to the fetus. The organisms spreading by transplacental route gain access to the maternal bloodstream in early infection. The intervillous space contains aggregates of (maternal) neutrophils admixed with fibrin in contrast to chronic villitis (Figure 6, 7). Acute villitis with marked microabscess formation and necrosis follows, since the trophoblast has receptors for the bacterial surface antigen internalin A, and cell-to-cell translocation of the bacteria across the placental barrier into the villous endothelial cells and fetal circulation occurs. Foci of acute intervillositis / villitis may coalesce to form punctate or confluent regions of abscess and necrosis that are grossly seen on placental sections.

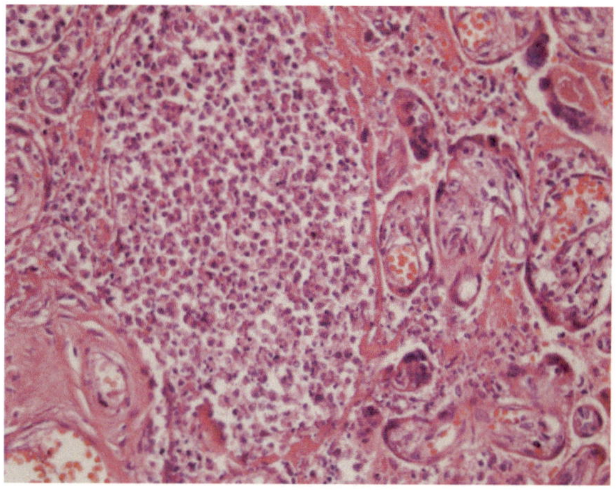

Figure 6. Acute villitis characterized by aggregates of neutrophils in the intervillous space admixed with fibrin.

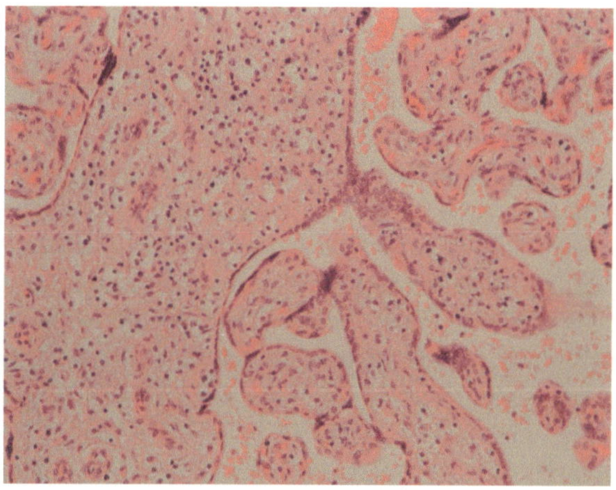

Figure 7. Acute villitis characterized by aggregates of neutrophils in the intervillous space admixed with fibrin.

Detection of acute villitis should prompt immediate notification of the perinatologists, since *Listeria monocytogenes* is a common cause and associated with rapid and disseminated fetal infection and high perinatal mortality in preterm births. This microorganism is a facultative anaerobe that can survive and replicate within a broad thermal range. Maternal infection is generally acquired through ingestion of contaminated food products (i.e. vegetables, packaged or refrigerated meats, dairy products). Tissue gram stains will show numerous, short gram positive rods. In addition, the placental lesions should be cultured, since investigations of perinatal death and epidemics may require detailed documentation through specific typing of the organism.

Other rare causes of acute villitis / intervillositis reflect maternal exposure to the pathogens. Acute fibrinopurulent inflammation due to *Chlamydia psittaci* will show organisms within syncytiotrophoblast. Maternal tularemia following tick bite, inhalation of airborne bacteria, or contact with infected rodents or rabbits can lead to a severe villitis and fetal infection. *Coccioides immitis* spherules produce an intense villitis / intervillositis but rarely transplacental infection of the fetus. Fetal sepsis due to *Escherichia coli* and group B and other streptococci can be evidenced by neutrophilia within the fetal chorionic villous capillaries that may infiltrate into the stroma forming aggregates in the subtrophoblastic space. In contrast to *L monocytogenes*, there is mild intervillositis or necrosis.

4.3. Chronic villitis

Chronic infections that may result in SPB are largely those caused by the TORCH (Toxoplasmosis, Others, Rubella virus, Cytomegalovirus, and Herpes simplex virus) infections. All of these infectious disease result in fetal onset of growth restriction, hepatosplenomegaly, cytopenias, coagulopathies, and often fetal hydrops and high infant morbidity and mortality. Parasitic pathogens are uncommon but may complicate gestations of women who have infected cats and are exposed early in their gestation to endemic pathogens. *Toxoplasma gondii* is the most important parasitic placental infection in Western countries [15].

The overwhelming majority (approximately 90%) of infectious chronic villitis is due to cytomegalovirus (CMV) and *Troponema pallidum* [16]. CMV infection usually results in a pale, hydropic-appearing placenta and preterm delivery frequently complicated by placental abruption. In these instances, dysmature villi are seen on light microscopy. More chronic infection generally results in a normal weight to shrunken, firm, pale, fibrotic placenta and fetal intrauterine growth restriction (IUGR). In these cases, CMV infection is characterized by lymphohistiocytic and especially, lymphoplasmacytic villitis. Plasma cell infiltrate, while not specific for CMV, is highly suggestive, especially if plasma cells are seen in terminal villi that are not in contiguity with the basal plate. Intranuclear or cytoplasmic trophoblastic epithelial, Hofbauer cellular, and endothelial inclusions are easily seen on hematoxylen eosin stains (Figure 8). However, immunoperoxidase stains for CMV are particularly useful in cases of longstanding intrauterine infection where the inclusions are sparse. Even if viral inclusions are unapparent; presence of stromal hemosiderin deposition due to capillary damage, dystrophic mineralization due to villous damage), and sclerosis are virtually pathognomonic of CMV. Lymphoplasmacytic deciduitis in the capsularis and basalis is generally present. Use of PCR for CMV early and late gene antigen gp 64 has also been reported [17].

Detection of acute villitis should prompt immediate notification of the perinatologists, since *Listeria monocytogenes* is a common cause and associated with rapid and disseminated fetal infection and high perinatal mortality in preterm births. This microorganism is a facultative anaerobe that can survive and replicate within a broad thermal range. Maternal infection is generally acquired through ingestion of contaminated food products (i.e. vegetables, packaged or refrigerated meats, dairy products). Tissue gram stains will show numerous, short gram positive rods.

Of special importance, prior maternal infection with CMV does not provide overall absolute immunity and therefore, most cases of congenital CMV are due to recurrent maternal infection that is asymptomatic in both the mother and the newborn. Since recurrent CMV is more

http://dx.doi.org/10.5772/54887

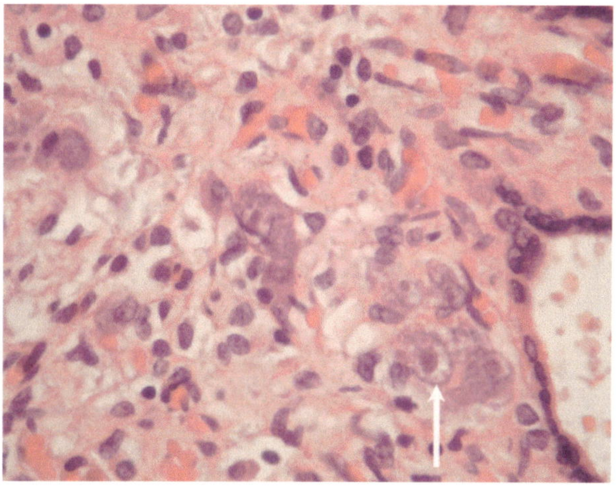

Figure 8. Intracytoplasmic inclusions (arrow) in a CMV villitis.

common than primary CMV infection during gestation, placental examination in SPB emerges as a critical means of detection of congenital CMV infection.

Syphilis placentitis is another cause of chronic villitis. The histopathology of *T pallidum* infection is T-lymphocytic and sometimes lymphoplasmacytic chronic villitis which are typically associated with sclerosis and circumferential vascular thickening of stem villous vessels and thrombosis. Sometimes, histopathology may be limited to villous edema and hypercellularity. Thrombi are also seen in umbilical cord and chorionic plate vessels, and confirmatory Warthin–Starry or Steiner silver stains are best performed on the umbilical cord because of its relative hypocellularity.

Herpes simplex virus (HSV) infection is characterized by lymphohistiocytic inflammation but marked necrosis and intervillositis with trophoblastic multinucleation and viral cytopathy. The villitis / intervillositis is similar to that seen in *L monocytogenes* except that the inflammation is more often chronic and trophoblastic glassy inclusions are present. Intranuclear inclusions can be confirmed by immunohistochemical stains. About 95% of intrauterine HSV infections are due to acute ascending infections from the maternal genital tract, and most occur with intact membranes. Therefore, amniotic multinucleation and necrosis is present, and frequently, lymphoplasmacytic chorioamnionitis. In more chronic cases these multinucleated residual cells may be incorporated into the superficial chorion. Chronic lymphoplasmacytic villitis is often accompanied by chronic deciduitis.

4.4. Idiopathic chronic deciduitis

Chronic deciduitis limited to the decidua basalis, and defined as diffuse lymphocytic infiltrate of the basal plate or any infiltrate in the decidua basalis that includes plasma cells is abnormal (Figure 9). It is suggested to represent maternal response to chronic intrauterine colonization or infection by organisms of low pathogenicity and may predispose to preterm birth. Potentially, infection may develop early in gestation, before membrane fusion of the chorioamnion of the gestational sac to the opposite uterine wall at 19–20 weeks, and then later after fusion, transmitted to the conceptus. Alternatively, the inflammation may represent recurrent / persistent low-grade infection that occurs between pregnancies as chronic endometritis. Therefore, it is a risk factor for recurrent pregnancy loss. In a study, it was found that 40% of preterm placentas from cases of idiopathic preterm labor and 15% of their control cases had chronic deciduitis [18]. Further clinicopathological studies may improve our understanding of the implications of this entity.

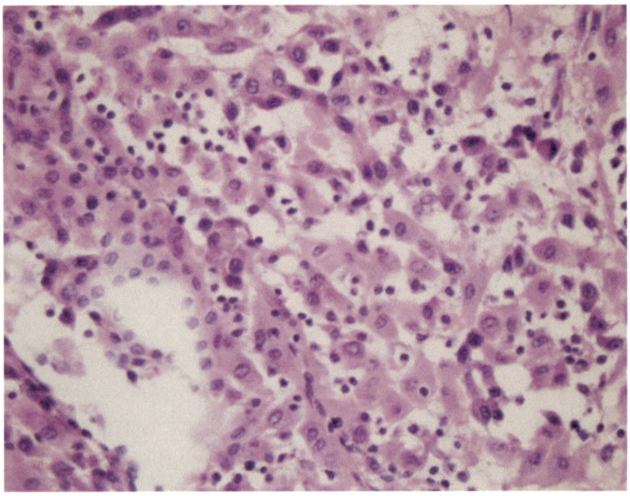

Figure 9. Chronic desiduitis including plasma cells in the decidua basalis.

5. Placental pathology of non-inflammatory processes in SPB

The pathogenesis of SPB in the absence of infection may also involve activation of pathways responsible for normal onset of labor via components of the maternal and fetal hypothalamic–pituitary–adrenal axis. These include loss of the normally coordinated interactions and changes in systemic and local uterine balances of oxytocin levels, fetal cortisol levels, and decreasing estrogen to progesterone ratios. Other non-infectious triggers of SPB are uteroplacental ischemia and / or oxidative stress, excessive uterine stretching, immunologically-mediated processes and uterine anomalies.

Finally, an important pathway also appears to involve non-infectious, pathological activation of decidual inflammation by decidual bleeding, because extravasated blood is a biochemical irritant and acts as a trigger of inflammation. Clinical findings suggest that pathological findings including chronic retromembraneous hemorrhage, marginal and retroplacental hematoma may have causal implications in SPB.

http://dx.doi.org/10.5772/54887

5.1. Chronic retromembranous hemorrhage

Gross examination of retromembraneous hemorrhage reveals marked discoloration characterized by red-brown thickenings and yellow areas behind the membranes, and opacity of the fetal surface (Figure 10). This lesion is most likely to be from old bleeding and ascending infection which are common together in extremely premature deliveries. The underlying cause of retromembranous hemorrhage may involve ischemia and / or endothelial damage. Decidua capsularis ischemia should be especially suspected if there is laminar necrosis or leukocytoclastic necrosis. In a recent study, immunohistochemical staining for some markers of oxidative stress including complement component 9 and nitrotyrosine residues were prominent in membrane rolls with laminar necrosis [19].

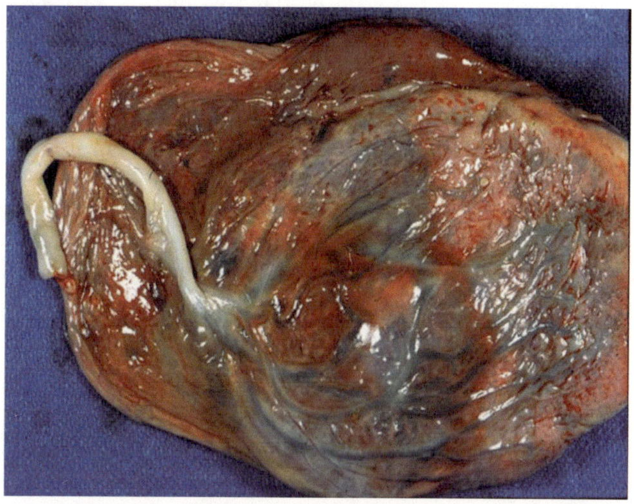

Figure 10. Retromembranous hemorrhages showing brown or yellow discolorations on the membranes.

In addition, tumor necrosis factor α (TNFα) production is a potential focus of ongoing researches on this topic, because TNFα in cervical secretions is of one of many potential cytokines that has been identified as a marker of preterm labor in women without risk factors of hypertension. It causes many effects and plays many roles on biological phenomena. TNFα production is a common outcome of activation of monocytes and histiocytes in tissue damage resulted from ischemia and bacteria, immune complexes, toxins and other cytokines TNFα causes the release of proteolytic enzymes from mesenchymal cells, in addition to resulting in aggregation and activation neutrophils. TNFα has also recently been shown to raise apoptosis of cultured villous trophoblasts [20]. Alternatively, it has a biological effect on inducing decidual vascular smooth muscle apoptosis and elastin degradation. TNFα also increases production of other inflammatory cytokines, matrix metalloproteinases involved in amnion degradation, and mediators of increased uterine tonicity (i.e., prostaglandin production by amnion, decidua and myometrium). Besides TNFα, other cytokines and chemokines such as IL-1β, IL-4, IL-6, IL-8 and factor Va are being investigated in preterm birth and seem to exhibit racial differences and polymorphisms, but their precise roles and points of entry in the cascade of preterm labor are unclear.

5.2. Retroplacental hematoma (Abruptio placenta)

Abruptio placenta is defined as the sudden separation of a significant portion of the placenta from its underlying maternal blood supply prior to delivery and is one important cause of acute hypoxic injury. It is associated with a number of adverse outcomes including preterm delivery, fetal growth restriction, stillbirth, and hypoxic ischemic encephalopathy. Patients with evidence of early pregnancy bleeding are also at risk for later acute abruption.

It is often stated that the correlation between pathological and clinical abruption is poor. Likewise, clinical signs and symptoms of abruption may also prove unreliable [21]. The gold standard for diagnosis of abruptio placenta is macroscopical appearance of retroplacental hemorrhage at the time of C-section. The best pathologic evidence is the gross finding of a retroplacental hematoma with either placental indentation or intraplacental extension (Figure 11). In the absence of these findings, microscopic evidence of interstitial hemorrhage in the basal plate or diffuse retromembranous hemorrhage is helpful to think about abruption. Ischemic changes in the overlying placenta such as recent villous infarction or villous stromal hemorrhage are also very suggestive of abruption. Finally, lesions associated with chronic maternal underperfusion are very commonly associated with abruption and can help strengthen a strong clinical suspicion of the diagnosis. Figure 12 illustrates morphological types of hemorrhagic and ischemic lesions of placental disk.

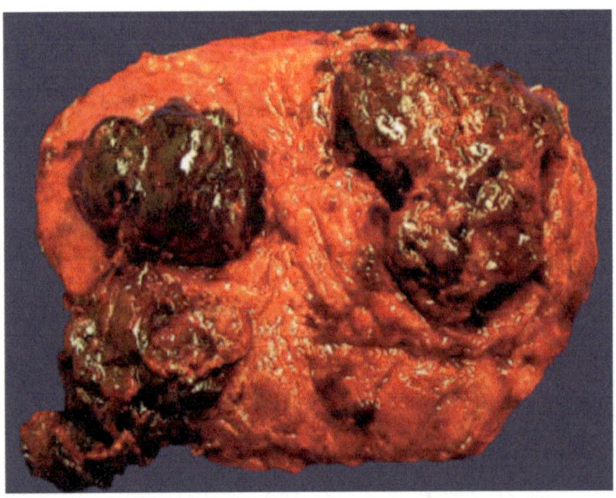

Figure 11. Gross appearance of the lesions of hematoma in the retroplacental area.

5.3. Marginal hematoma

Chronic marginal hematoma (chronic abruption) is an important cause of preterm delivery and may be associated with an atypical form of neonatal lung disease. It is also a significant risk factor for cerebral palsy and other forms of worse neurological outcome in term infants.

http://dx.doi.org/10.5772/54887

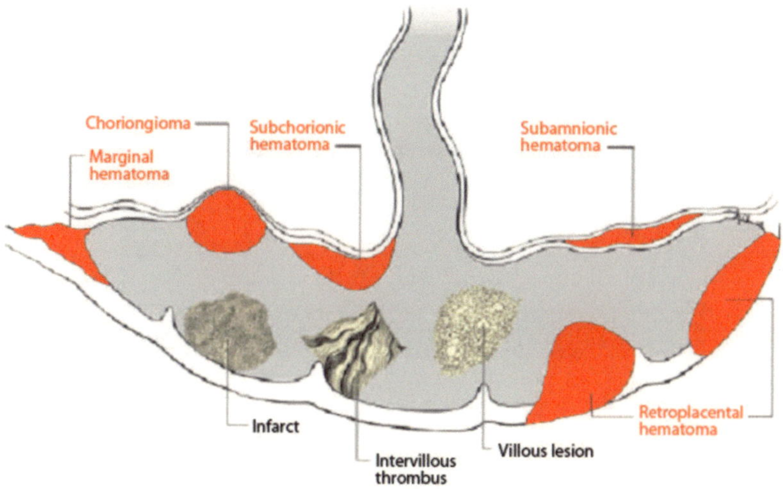

Figure 12. Morphological illustration of placental hemorrhagic and ischemic lesions.

Factors that have been associated with chronic abruption include multiparity, smoking, oligohydramnios, and excessively deep uterine implantation.

Unlike arterial rupture resulting in abruptio placenta, venous hemorrhage tends to occur at the placental margins and to escape at lower pressure in chronic abruption. Therefore, in contrast to retroplacental hematoma, hemorrhage of lower pressure accumulation plays a role in the process of preterm labor. The pathogenetic explanation is that lateral growth of the placenta involves remodeling of large uterine veins and these large obliquely oriented structures may rupture prematurely if poorly supported by the surrounding endometrium or subjected to elevated intramural pressure due to obstruction of larger upstream veins such as the vena cava. For these reasons, marginal abruptions may not result in immediate delivery, instead acute form presents as threatened abortion in early pregnancy or chronic abruption occurs in later pregnancy causing bleeding with preterm birth or spontaneous abortion, if it shows rapidly enlarging of great enough volume or recurs. Additionally, chronic abruption is often associated with oligohydramnios in a syndrome known as the chronic abruption-oligohydramnios sequence.

Clinically, marginal hematoma may be seen on prenatal ultrasonogram and is referred to as subchorionic hemorrhage or periplacental hemorrhage. They may be detected early in gestation and resolve later and lead to circumvallation. It is important to note that the clinically

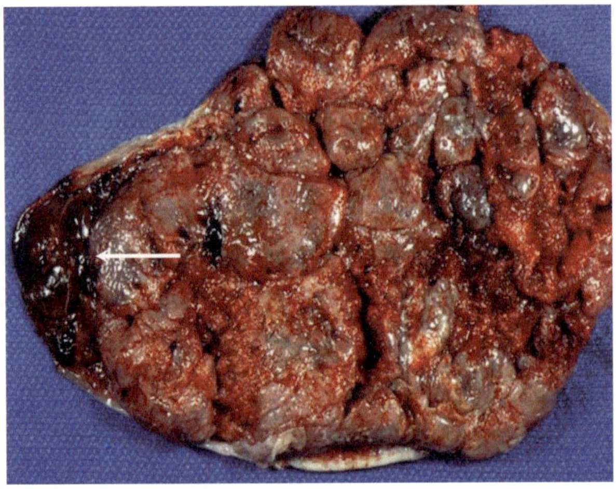

Figure 13. Marginal hematoma extending onto the membranes (white arrow). The brown color of the blood indicates its chronicity.

used term "subchorionic hemorrhage" is different from "subchorionic thrombohematoma", also called Breus mole, which refers to a central, nodular protuberance on the fetal surface of the placenta, and from thrombohematoma formation in the maternal space.

Examination of suspected marginal hematoma should include recording of its dimensions and percentage of marginal involvement, type of adherence and appearance, features of chronicity, extent of dissection of adjacent parenchyma on section, and type of associated, overlying membranous insertion, along with histological evaluation of the junctional region and membranes. They are crescent-shaped and have a cut surface with a triangular configuration at the lateral angle of the placenta (Figure 13). There is associated dissection into the lateral chorionic villous parenchyma. Chronic form may produce a depression in adjacent marginal chorionic villous tissue. On section, it has a laminated, friable, yellowish-brown and / or calcified thrombohematoma with dissection of the lateral placental border. A superimposed acute component may be also present.

Chronic abruption, like chronic maternal underperfusion, is associated with a cluster of placental findings. These include old marginal blood clot, circumvallate membrane insertion, chorioamnionic hemosiderin deposition, and green (biliverdin) staining of the fetal surface *Circumvallation* may develop as a consequence of blood accumulating in the space between the decidua and chorion leading to folding of the marginal chorionic plate. When circumvallation is attributable to chronic marginal separation, old blood clot and local *hemosiderin deposition* are seen on histological sections. Hemosiderin stains blue by iron stain, but other hemoglobin related pigments do not. Any pigment seen in a premature placenta favors chronic abruption rather than meconium release which is extremely uncommon before 37 weeks. Additionally, the finding of hemosiderosis in the decidua basalis should always be documented, but when seen in cases of SPB in the absence of a clinical history of maternal hypertension, it may have different implications and reflect a genetic or ethnic risk factor.

To be noted, marginal hematomas are often acute and affect less than a quadrant of the placental perimeter. They are reportedly seen in 0.7–1.9% of placentas [22]. This percentage may relatively increase in the academic tertiary units where large numbers of patients are admitted for complicated gestations and SPB. In a study, therefore, incidence of chronic marginal hematoma was found in 7–10% of placentas [7].

Incidental marginal hematoma or passive, intrapartum accumulation of blood in the marginal anatomic fissure, with no grossly detectable loss of the distinct border between the lateral placental margin and the borders of the hematoma, may accompany oxytocin induction, such as seen in IPB.

6. Placental pathology in induced preterm birth

Induction of labor with or without artificial rupture of membranes, and caesarean section delivery in cases of IPB is largely performed for maternal hypertensive disorders of pregnancy, non-reassuring fetal heart rate and IUGR.

The pathology of the spectrum of pregnancy induced hypertensive conditions as they relate to IUGR and the placental pathology associated with IUGR may be seen in preterm and term placentas [23]. The other disorders that predispose to maternal indications for IPB are also largely related to those that result in chronic uteroplacental underperfusion and risk of IUGR, such as vasculopathy and thrombosis associated with maternal primary hypertension or diabetes mellitus (maternal vascular obstructive lesions). Thus, there is some overlap between maternal and fetal indications for indicated preterm delivery. However, there are some placental pathologies that may not be associated with IUGR but with fetal distress in the preterm birth, and some that have been found to be causally linked to IUGR, non-reassuring fetal heart rate, and / or absent umbilical arterial end diastolic blood flow. The following entities are more likely seen in placentas from induced or caesarean section deliveries performed for fetal indications, and that might be expected to be identified in different frequencies in late versus early preterm placentas.

7. Chronic uteroplacental underperfussion

Chronically underperfused placentas are associated with fetal growth restriction, preterm birth due to either premature labor or premature rupture of membranes, premature placental separation (abruptio placenta), and carry an increased risk for the development of preeclampsia. Clinical conditions predisposing to maternal underperfusion include type I diabetes mellitus, connective tissue disease, chronic renal insufficiency, essential hypertension, and underlying maternal coagulopathies including thrombophilic mutations and antiphospholipid syndrome. Familial aggregation of preeclampsia and underlying maternal vascular disease may at least in part be due inheritance of the so-called metabolic syndrome characterized by abnormal serum lipid levels, enhanced production of acute phase inflammatory mediators, and a predisposition to vascular damage related to reactive oxygen intermediates.

Chronic maternal underperfusion of the intervillous space can result from a variety of causes including underlying cardiac insufficiency, failure to expand intravascular volume during pregnancy, or structural abnormalities in arteries supplying the uterus. It is currently believed that the major process leading to underperfusion is failure of trophoblast to appropriately invade and remodel the uterine spiral arteries. While the exact mechanisms of events leading to this outcome have not yet been explained, but a number of contributing factors have been identified. These include initial exposure to fetoplacental antigens in the first pregnancies, inherited polymorphisms in genes of the renin-angiotensin system, circulating anti-endothelial cell antibodies, and underlying uterine small vessel disease. The common activator for all of these factors seems to be decreased oxygen delivery to the implantation site resulting in impaired trophoblast differentiation and inadequate placentation. In the absence of arterial remodeling, the placenta is chronically underperfused leading to decreased fetoplacental growth and, in some cases, release of vasoactive mediators in late pregnancy leading to the clinical syndrome of preeclampsia.

Placentas affected by maternal underperfusion generally show multiple pathological findings that together allow a specific diagnosis to be rendered. One important, often overlooked, feature is decreased body weight for gestational age and decreased placental weight relative to that of the infant, which suggests increased fetoplacental weight ratio. In severe cases, this correlates with late impairment of placental growth (distal villous hypoplasia) as the fetus sacrifices placental perfusion in order to supply critical vascular beds such as the central nervous and cardiovascular systems. Also common in severe cases are villous infarcts caused by thrombosis of abnormal maternal arteries and a thin umbilical cord resulting from extracellular volume depletion and decreased hydration of Wharton's jelly. Lesser degrees or durations of underperfusion and hypoxia can lead to stasis with intervillous fibrin deposition, accelerated syncytiotrophoblast turnover with increased syncytial knots, and ischemia leading to foci of villous agglutination (Figure 14). Finally, there are other findings directly reflecting inadequate placentation. These include muscularization of basal plate arteries, aggregates of immature or prematurely differentiated cells such as placental site giant cells or epithelioid (chorion laeve type) trophoblasts in the basal plate, and medial hypertrophy or fibrinoid necrosis (acute atherosis) of maternal arterioles in the membranous decidua (Figure 15).

8. Chronic villitis of unknown etiology

Villitis of unknown etiology (VUE) represents a subcategory of chronic villitis and has not been proven clinically or identified histopathologically to result from an infection in the placenta, mother or infant [24]. VUE is a common lymphohistiocytic villitis affecting terminal villi with vasculosyncytial membrane formation which is a characteristic morphological feature of 32 or more weeks of gestational development. Therefore, the diagnosis should be restricted to the cases of 32–36 weeks.

http://dx.doi.org/10.5772/54887

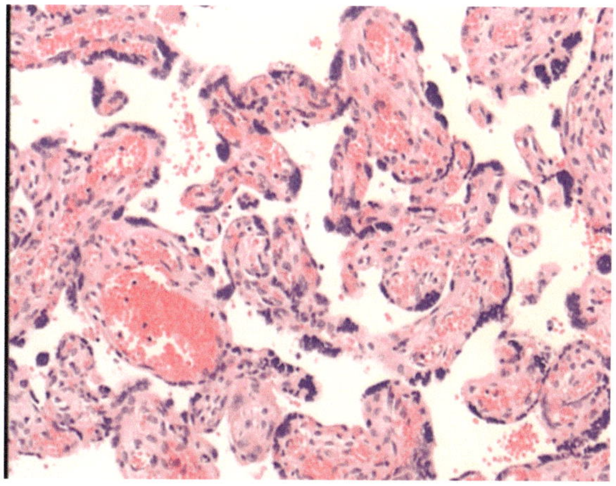

Figure 14. Histopathological features in placentas affected by maternal underperfusion including increased syncytial knots due to increased apoptosis and accelerated syncytiotrophoblast turnover.

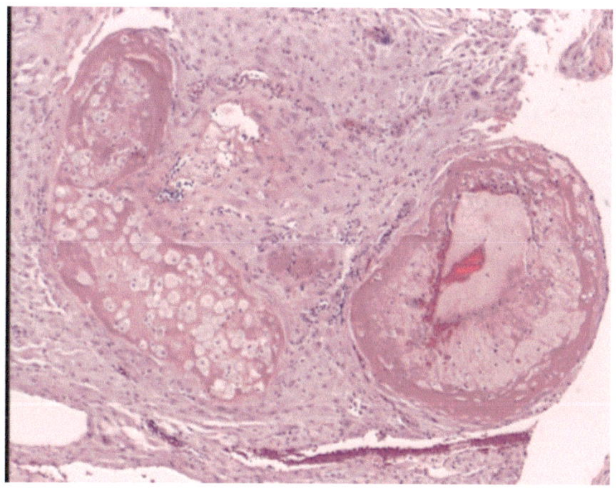

Figure 15. Endothelial damage in maternal underperfusion characterized by medial hypertrophy or fibrinoid necrosis (acute atherosis).

VUE does not have consistent gross pathological features. Because of its irregular distribution, the histological detection of VUE is sample-dependent. It is best detected at low power magnification (20×), typically in the subchorionic and especially basal villi. Higher power view generally reveals lymphohistiocytic villitis affecting less than five villi (Figure 16). Plasma cells are rarely seen, but depending on the stage, the villitis may be accompanied by villous destruction, sclerosis, and the very rarely giant cell reaction. Lymphoplasmacytic deciduitis of the basal plate and chronic chorioamnionitis characterized by foci of small lymphocytic infiltrates in the lower chorion may be also seen. If the villous inflammation is patchy and involves more than 5% of chorionic villi, it is termed "diffuse VUE". In diffuse form the midzonal parenchyma is generally not spared, perivillous fibrin deposition is seen, and villous destruction is more prominent.

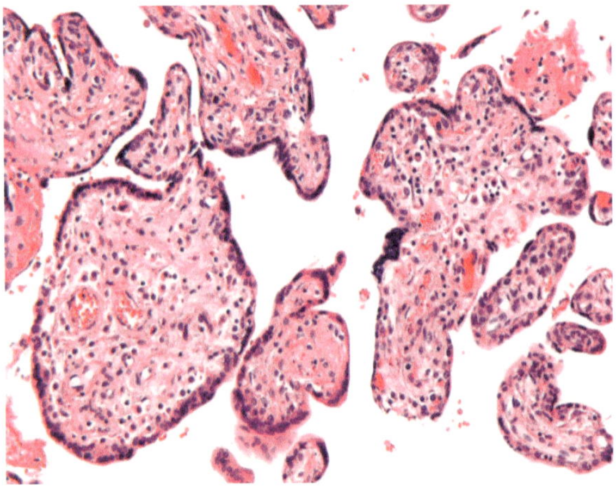

Figure 16. Lymphohistiocytic villitis in a case of preterm birth with VUE.

Most cases of VUE do not result in perinatal morbidity and mortality. However, there is a strong risk correlation between VUE and idiopathic IUGR. The frequency of IUGR directly correlates with the diffuse form. VUE has also been shown to be linked to non-infectious spontaneous preterm birth and perinatal asphyxia [25]. The presence of VUE may contribute to placental insufficiency and to the oligohydramnios without a maternal hypertensive disorder or other risk factor. Diffuse VUE with an inflammatory involvement of larger stem villi and villous vessels, termed "chronic villitis with obliterative vasculopathy", is also more strongly associated with severe IUGR and perinatal morbidity, including neurological sequelae.

The most important pathogenetic characteristic of VUE is that it appears to represent a localized, alloimmune process of host versus graft response in the chorionic villous tree from a breakdown in maternal–fetal tolerance. The lymphohistiocytic villous infiltrates have been shown to be composed almost exclusively of maternal CD8-positive T cells and Hofbauer cells of fetal origin. Activation of fetal Hofbauer cells and focal syncytiotrophoblast destruction at sites of villitis, together with the absence of eosinophils and presence of histiocytic giant cells are compatible with a delayed hypersensitivity response or a T-helper 1 type of response. The hypothesis that VUE is an alloimmune-mediated process is supported by its high risk of recurrence (10–25%) and 60% rate of pregnancy loss in instances of recurrence.

Massive chronic intervillositis (MCI) is also an alloimmune phenomenon, but it is unclear if it is a variant of VUE. MCI is most frequently seen in first trimester abortion, and therefore might be expected to be more prevalent in placentas from extremely and severely preterm birth It is also a potential cause of IUGR in the preterm infant in IPB or non-infectious SPB. (Figure 17)

http://dx.doi.org/10.5772/54887

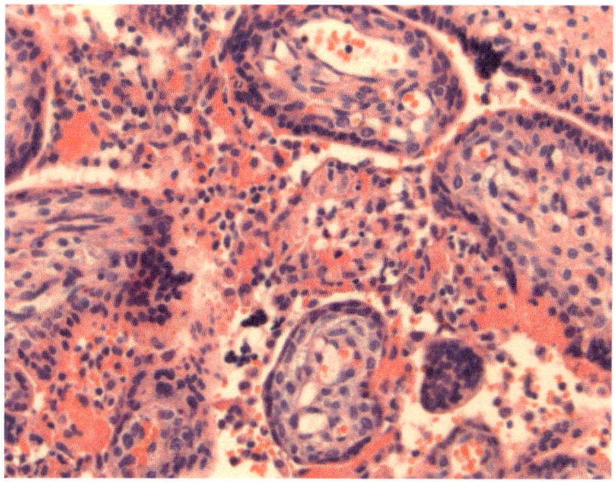

Figure 17. Histiocytic intervillitis in an extremely preterm birth complicated by mortality.

9. Fetal thrombotic vasculopathy

Fetal thrombotic vasculopathy (FTV) is explained by the biological fact that vessels of the chorionic villous tree are in continuity with those in the fetus. The presence of chorionic villous thrombi leads to fetal thromboembolic phenomena and increased placental vascular resistance, and may lead to loss of end-diastolic blood flow, which may exacerbate any underlying cord or fetal factors that predispose to thrombosis.

Thromboocclusive lesions of large fetal vessels in the placenta and umbilical cord occur in the context of one or more of the classic triad of risk factors; vascular stasis, loss of surface resistance to coagulation, and circulatory hypercoagulability. Possible causes of fetal vascular stasis include prolonged umbilical cord obstruction, increased central venous pressure, and elevated hematocrit. Loss of surface resistance to coagulation may occur with severe fetal inflammation, antiphospholipid syndrome, and other forms of vessel wall damage. Circulatory hypercoagulability may be present with platelet disorders, maternal diabetes, or thrombophilic mutations involving protein C, protein S, antithrombin II, factor V, prothrombin 2010, and methyl tetrahydrofolate reductase. It is likely that most cases of fetal thromboocclusive disease involve more than one risk factor.

Sustained proximal vascular occlusion leads to degenerative changes in the distal villous tree. Longstanding occlusion of large arteries leads to distal hyalinized avascular villi. The early stages of proximal venous occlusion cause circulatory stasis with villous stromal-vascular karyorrhexis which is degeneration of red blood cells, endothelial cells, and villous stromal fibroblasts. This pattern of change occurs diffusely in the placentas of stillbirths. When seen in a focal distribution in either live births or stillborns it has been termed hemorrhagic endovasculitis. With longstanding venous obstruction, upstream villi become hyalinized and avascular as with arterial obstruction. These villous changes can affect large or small groups of villi and can be localized or widely distributed throughout the placental parenchyma. When the number of affected villi exceeds an average of ≥ 15 villi/ slide the process has been termed fetal thrombotic vasculopathy (Figure 18). Large vessel thrombi are identified in approximately one third of such cases. Other lesions associated with fetal thrombo-occlusive disease include intimal fibrin cushions and fibromuscular sclerosis of stem arteries (Figure 19). Intimal fibrin cushions are intramural aggregates of fibrin in proximal fetal veins that are usually attributed to increased intramural pressure. Fibromuscular sclerosis represents concentric narrowing of the vascular lumen by proliferating smooth muscle cells and subendothelial fibroblasts, typically occurring in placental vessels lying between the point of occlusion and the affected villi secondary to lack of flow.

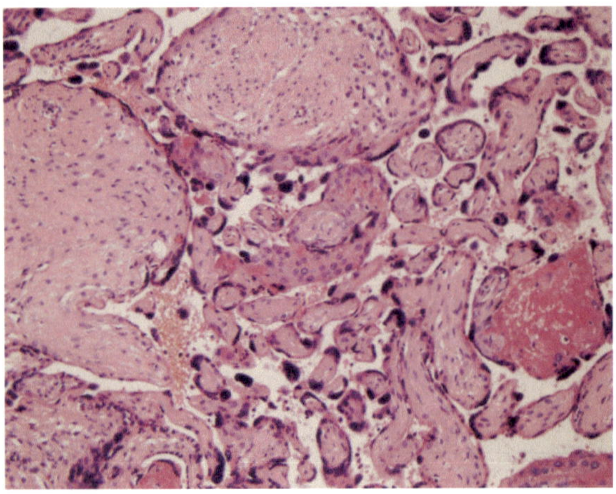

Figure 18. Avascular villi associated with fetal thrombo-occlusive disease.

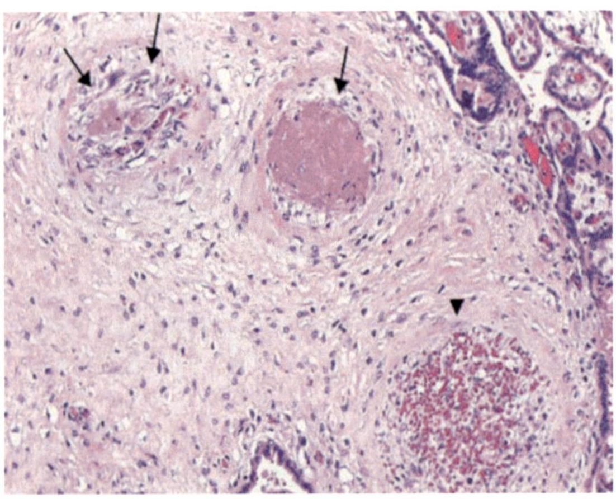

Figure 19. Intimal fibrin cushions and fibromuscular sclerosis of stem arteries, a suggestive histological finding for fetal thrombo-occlusive disease.

FTV is a significant risk factor for thromboembolic neurological sequelae such as a stroke. Other thromboembolic sequelae include limb reduction anomalies, systemic visceral thromboemboli in the gastrointestinal tract, kidneys, and liver. Hepatic thrombosis may lead to Budd–Chiari syndrome and perinatal liver disease. IUGR with FTV is likely related to loss of functional placental parenchyma. Avascular villi are also associated with IUGR, chronic monitoring abnormalities, and discordant growth in twin gestations. Nonocclusive thrombi in severely inflamed chorionic vessels are occasionally seen with severe acute chorioamnionitis in very low birth weight infants and represent a risk factor for neurologic impairment in this subgroup.

10. Maternal floor infarction

Maternal floor infarction (MFI) is also associated with high rates of preterm birth (26–60%) and unexplained IUGR (24–100%) [26]. When it shows an early onset, there is an associated increased risk of recurrence and severity in subsequent pregnancies. The dense perivillous fibrinoid deposition impairs villous exchange resulting in villous atrophy. The etiopathogenesis of the perivillous accumulation of fibrinoid in MFI is likely complex, but there is good evidence that it may be immune mediated.

11. Conclusion

Preterm birth is common and is associated with high rates of perinatal morbidity and mortality. Pathological examination of the preterm placenta can provide valuable information concerning the immediate and chronic risks for the infant and risks of chronic diseases in childhood.

The gross and microscopic examination of the placenta from preterm birth, whenever possible, should be approached with the clinical perspective of whether the specimen is from an SPB or IPB. Placentas from SPB more commonly show acute chorioamnionitis with funisitis and intense vasculitis, marginal hematoma, chronic decidual hemorrhage, and acute and chronic infectious villitis. SPB due to POL and / or PPROM likely results from abnormal activation a cascade of cellular components and mediators of an inflammatory pathway are responsible for the process of normal, term parturition. Placentas from IPB more commonly show fetal thrombotic vasculopathy. Diffuse VUE and chronic villitis with obliterative vasculopathy are very common in late IPB, whereas those from early IPB show chronic intervillositis more frequently. All of these diagnoses have implications for the neonate and/or the mother.

Further studies may reveal that maternal chorionic villous inflammatory cells, as seen in syphilis and toxoplasmosis, play a role in many other infectious villitides and that the effects of these cells contribute to the severity of the morbidity or mortality that has been largely attributed to the infectious organisms. Research may also reveal that the maternal lymphocytes in VUE and even infections may gain access to fetal circulation. The prolonged period that a mother's lymphocytes may be in her child's circulation may have implications for the etiologies of other pediatric immune-mediated disorders. FTV may also predispose the infant to short or long term persistence of increased vascular tone or vascular disease, in addition to functional deficiencies of major organs such as the liver or kidneys.

Thus, the placenta in preterm birth is not only a record of adverse conditions during intrauterine life that led to SPB or necessitated an IPB, it also likely holds clues to predicting which individuals will be at heightened risks for developing chronic diseases in childhood. Low birth weight infants are at risk for developing chronic diseases in adulthood. Pathological examination of the preterm placenta may provide important insights into future investigations to determine which infants will be at risk for development of cardiovascular disease, hypertension and diabetes mellitus, later in life. Risks of neurological sequelae in the infant have been linked to specific histopathological features in the placenta. The placental pathology report should include notation of these features.

In conclusion, placental pathologists are in a unique position to provide valuable observations in preterm birth. Their service in the perinatal medicine;

- may provide an immediate impact on the care of the premature newborn,
- may help to explain the poorly understood pathogenetic mechanisms responsible for preterm birth,
- and may potentially aid in the process of linking currently unexplained roles of alloimmune-mediated processes and intrauterine stress to the development of chronic human diseases.

Author details

Erdener Ozer

Address all correspondence to: erdener.ozer@deu.edu.tr

Department of Pathology, Dokuz Eylul University School of Medicine, Izmir, Turkey

References

[1] Goldenberg RL, Culhane JF, Iams JD, et al. Epidemiology and causes of preterm birth. Lancet 2008;371:75–84.

[2] World Health Organization. Media Center: Preterm Birth, Fact Sheet. http://www.who.int/mediacentre/factsheets/fs363/en/index.html (accessed 1 October 2012).

[3] Alexander JM, Gilstrap LC, Cox SM, et al. Clinical chorioamnionitis and the prognosis for very low birth weight infants. Obstetrics and Gynecology 1998;91:725–729.

[4] Romero R, Espinoza J, Goncalves LF, et al. The role of inflammation and infection in preterm birth. Seminars in Reproductive Medicine 2007;25:21–39.

[5] Goldenberg RL, Andrews WW, Goepfert AR, et al. The Alabama Preterm Birth Study: umbilical cord blood Ureaplasma urealyticum and Mycoplasma hominis cultures in very preterm newborn infants. American Journal of Obstetrics and Gynecology 2008;198:e41–45.

[6] Steel JH, Malatos S, Kennea N, et al. Bacteria and inflammatory cells in fetal membranes do not always cause preterm labor. Pediatrics Research 2005;57:404–411.

[7] Redline RW. Placental pathology: a systematic approach with clinical correlations. Placenta 2008;29(suppl A):S86–91.

[8] Arias F, Victoria A, Cho K, Kraus F. Placental histology and clinical characteristics of patients with preterm premature rupture of membranes. Obstetrics and Gynecology 1997;89:265-271.

[9] Redline R, Faye-Petersen O, Heller D, et al. Amniotic infection syndrome: nosology and reproducibility of placental reaction patterns. Pediatric and Developmental Pathology 2003; 6: 435-48

[10] Benirschke KKP, Baergen RN. Pathology of the human placenta. New York: Springer; 2006.

[11] 47 Kraus FT, Redline RW, Gersell DJ, et al. Placental Pathology. In: Atlas of Nontumor Pathology. Washington, DC: Armed Forces Institute of Pathology, American Registry of Pathology; 2004:p75–115.

[12] Redline RW. Inflammatory responses in the placenta and umbilical cord. Seminars in Fetal and Neonatal Medicine 2006;11:296–301.

[13] Qureshi F, Jacques SM, Bendon RW, et al. Candida funisitis: a clinicopathologic study of 32 cases. Pediatric and Developmental Pathology 1998;1:118–124.

[14] Ohyama M, Itani Y, Yamanaka M, et al. Re-evaluation of chorioamnionitis and funisitis with a special reference to subacute chorioamnionitis. Human Pathology 2002;33:183–190.

[15] Fowler KB, Stagno S, Pass RF, et al. The outcome of congenital cytomegalovirus infection in relation to maternal antibody status. New England Journal of Medicine 1992;326:663–667.

[16] Redline RW. Villitis of unknown etiology: noninfectious chronic villitis in the placenta. Human Pathology 2007;38:1439–1446.

[17] Nakamura Y, Sakuma S, Ohta Y, et al. Detection of the human cytomegalovirus gene in placental chronic villitis by polymerase chain reaction. Human Pathology 1994;25:815–818.

[18] Edmondson N, Bocking A, Machin G, et al. The prevalence of chronic deciduitis in cases of preterm labour without clinical chorioamnionitis. Pediatric and Developmental Pathology 2009;12:16-21.

[19] Stanek J, Al-Ahmadie HA. Laminar necrosis of placental membranes: a histologic sign of uteroplacental hypoxia. Pediatric and Developmental Pathology 2005;8:34–42.

[20] Menon R, Camargo MC, Thorsen P, et al. Amniotic fluid interleukin-6 increase is an indicator of spontaneous preterm birth in white but not black Americans. American Journal of Obstetrics and Gynecology 2008;198:e71–77.

[21] Ananth CV, Wilcox AJ. Placental abruption and perinatal mortality in the United States. American Journal of Epidemiology 2001;153:332-337.

[22] Fox HSN, Sebire NJ. Pathology of the Placenta. In: Major Problems in Pathology. Philadelphia: Saunders Elsevier; 2007:p123–337.

[23] Salafia CM, Charles AK, Maas EM. Placenta and fetal growth restriction. Clinics in Obstetrics and Gynecology 2006;49:236-256.

[24] Jacques SM, Qureshi F. Chronic villitis of unknown etiology in twin gestations. Pediatric Pathology 1994;14:575-584.

[25] Bjoro K Jr, Myhre E. The role of chronic non-specific inflammatory lesions of the placenta in intra-uterine growth retardation. Acta Pathologica Microbiologica et Immunologica Scandinavica 1984;92:133–137.

[26] Faye-Petersen OM, Heller DS, Joshi VV. Handbook of Placental Pathology. Oxford: Taylor and Francis; 2006.

Section 2

Short and Long Term Effect of Preterm Birth

Chapter 5

Microbes and the Inflammatory Response in Necrotising Enterocolitis

Heather J.L. Brooks, Michelle A. McConnell and
Roland S. Broadbent

Additional information is available at the end of the chapter

http://dx.doi.org/10.5772/55039

1. Introduction

Necrotising enterocolitis (NEC) is a progressive disease of the neonatal intestine beginning in the distal ileum and proximal colon and characterised by inflammatory necrosis [1,2]. It typically affects low birth-weight, preterm infants who account for the majority (70–90%) of cases [3–5]. Since the 1960s, advances in medical care have raised the survival rate for preterm infants with increasingly shortened gestation periods, resulting in a concomitant surge in NEC cases. The overall incidence of NEC is generally accepted as ranging from <1% to 5% of neonatal intensive care unit (NICU) admissions, or up to 5 cases per 1,000 live births [4–6]. There is an inverse relationship between NEC and birth-weight, so that very low birth-weight infants (VLBW; <1500 g) carry the greatest burden of disease [4,5,7]. Caplan reported NEC rates for VLBW infants vary greatly across countries, ranging from 1.5% in Japan to 28% in Hong Kong, with racial disparity apparent in VLBW black infants who have an increased risk and greater associated mortality [5,8]. Despite advances in neonatal care, the overall mortality remains high at around 20–30% [3,8-10]. An estimated 20-40% of infants with NEC require surgery, which has a case fatality rate of up to 50%, the smallest, least mature infants having the worst prognosis [5]. Most cases of NEC are sporadic with no clear seasonal distribution, but outbreaks have been documented [5]. Treatment of NEC is mainly supportive with the administration of broad-spectrum antibiotics while surgery is indicated for intestinal perforation or removal of necrotic bowel segments. NEC complications and sequelae include serious neurodevelopmental delay, poor growth, intestinal obstruction due to scarring, short bowel syndrome, and liver failure due to prolonged hyperalimentation [6, 9]. The annual financial cost of NEC is considerable and in the USA has been estimated at $500 million to $1 billion [9].

1.1. Clinical classification

The classification system of Bell has historically proved important in defining three main stages: suspected, definite and advanced NEC [11]. Modifications to Bell's criteria have provided a more detailed system of clinical staging as shown in Table 1 [12,13]. However, Gordon et al and others have challenged the belief that NEC is a single entity, preferring to view it as an umbrella term for a number of separate diseases with some common features [13,14]. Although relatively uncommon, conditions, which mimic neonatal NEC, such as focal bowel perforation, intussusception, ecchymotic colitis, appendicitis and shigellosis, have been reported and may complicate the clinical diagnosis [14-18].

Stage (NEC)	Systemic signs	Radiographic findings	Intestinal signs
Stage I (suspected)	Temperature instability, apnoea, bradycardia	Normal or intestinal dilation; mild ileus	Gastric residuals, occult blood, mild abdominal distension
Stage II A (definite)	Temperature instability, apnoea, bradycardia	Intestinal dilation, ileus, focal pneumatosis	Blood in stools, prominent abdominal distension, absent bowel sounds
Stage II B (definite)	As above plus mild metabolic acidosis and thrombocytopenia	As II A plus portal vein gas, ascites	Abdominal wall oedema with palpable loops and tenderness
Stage III A (advanced)	As stage II B plus mixed acidosis, oligouria, hypotension, coagulopathy	As II B plus worsening ascites	Worsening wall oedema, erythema and induration
Stage III B (advanced)	As II A, shock, deterioration in vital signs	As II B plus pneumoperitoneum	Perforated bowel

Table 1. Modified Bell's staging for necrotising enterocolitis (adapted from Kliegman RM et al and Gordon et al [12,13])

1.2. Risk factors

So far, four major risk factors for NEC have been defined with prematurity being the most consistent. At 36 weeks gestation there is a sharp decrease in the incidence of NEC, supporting the concept that gut maturation provides significant protection against development of the disease [4]. Nevertheless, NEC in term and high birth-weight infants is not unknown, although the risk factors appear to be somewhat different [4,6,13]. The introduction of enteral feeds, particularly formula milk, and subsequent colonisation of the neonatal intestinal tract with bacteria are believed to be significant risk factors in the development of NEC [4,6,19]. Not only does formula milk lack the gastrointestinal protective, anti-inflammatory and maturation factors present in breast milk, it can be a source of *Cronobacter sakazakii*, a neonatal pathogen implicated in some cases of NEC [19]. Early research concentrated on the role of hypoxia and ischaemia, with the idea that the subsequent mucosal injury due to lack of oxygenation initiates NEC through promotion of bacterial translocation and the inflammatory cascade [1]. Many animal models of NEC have subsequently relied on reproducing this type of damage [5,20,21]. Kosloske et al suggested the 'dive reflex', whereby blood flow is diverted away from the GI tract to vital organs, as one mechanism of intestinal injury but current opinion, based on analyses of risk factors over several decades, favours a secondary role for hypoxia-ischaemia [5]. Nevertheless, the fact that NEC most commonly occurs in the distal ileum and proximal colon, the watershed areas of the mesenteric arteries, suggests inadequate or disordered blood circulation constitutes a risk factor in some circumstances [1,22]. Prenatal circulatory events, umbilical and aortic catheterisation with dispersion of small emboli and congenital heart disease have been linked to NEC, but occur in a minority of cases [2,4]. Preterm neonates are more susceptible to hypoxia and intestinal ischaemia than term neonates because of poor vascular resistance [1,4,22]. However, there is a stronger association between NEC, prematurity, enteral feeding and the presence of bacteria in the GI tract than hypoxia-ischaemia [1,5,22]. Overall, ischaemia/reperfusion injury seems to be more relevant to the development of NEC in term infants and those preterm infants with spontaneous intestinal perforations [23]. Yet hypoxia may exert a subtle effect by sensitising the intestinal epithelium to bacterial products and this is discussed in more detail in section 4.1 [24].

Recent evidence has linked blood transfusions with subsequent NEC in extremely premature infant [25–30]. The terms TANEC (Transfusion Associated NEC) and TRAGI (Transfusion-Related Acute Gut Injury) have been coined, referring to this association [25,31]. A recent meta-analysis examining evidence for the association concludes that recent transfusion is associated with NEC, and that transfusion-associated NEC has a higher risk of mortality than NEC which was not preceded by transfusion [25]. The reason for the association, and whether it is causal has not been elucidated. Prior to concern about TRAGI, Doppler studies have shown a decrease in neonatal superior mesenteric blood flow during and after blood transfusion [32]. The reason for this is not clear, but blood transfusion appears to have wide-ranging effects on haemodynamics, possibly as a result of changes in the microcirculation. Digestion of food requires a major increase in gut blood supply and it has been suggested that limiting or ceasing milk feeds before, during and after a blood transfusion in susceptible babies may decrease the risk of TRAGI. This has not been subjected to any systematic study and therefore remains speculative. The need for a co-ordinated approach to investigate the association between blood transfusion and NEC has been highlighted by Blau et al and there is an online world registry for TRAGI (www.tragiregistry.com) [31]. Any trial of an intervention for TRAGI prophylaxis would need large numbers, requiring a multicentre approach.

There are other characteristics of the preterm infant favouring the development of NEC. The combination of poor gut motility and under-production of mucous decreases clearance and increases exposure of the epithelium to potentially harmful components of the luminal contents [1,5,19]. Moreover, induction of foetal hypoxia can further reduce postnatal intestinal motility [1]. The lumen contents of preterm infants may be more acidic, due to inadequate digestion/absorption of nutrients and bacterial fermentation of undigested milk, or more toxic, as formula feeding elicits toxic bile acids [1]. Bacterial overgrowth, as indicated by a positive hydrogen breath test, is considered to be a further consequence of delayed transit time and may promote NEC through increasing bacterial translocation from the intestinal lumen into the tissues or through exposure to high concentrations of bacterial antigens [33,34]. More recently, it has been proposed that genetic polymorphisms in the genes encoding the interleukin (IL) 4 binding receptor alpha chain and the chemokine IL-8 may also be a risk factor for NEC [35]. Intrauterine infection is another risk factor for NEC; the microorganisms implicated and proposed causality are discussed in section 2.3.

In the normal course of events, acquisition of the enteric microbiota begins during the birth process through the ingestion of bacteria of maternal origin. Breastfeeding, handling by the mother and exposure to environmental bacteria create further opportunities for gaining new species [6]. Colonisation takes place in the first few days of life and is influenced by a multitude of factors such as mode of delivery, type of feeding (breast milk or formula), gestation age, hospitalisation, the surrounding environs, maternal infection and antibiotic therapy, with mode of delivery and type of feeding considered the most significant [36]. Whereas breast fed infants are regarded as having an enteric microbiota rich in bifidobacteria, a more diverse microbiota, including potentially pathogenic groups such as *Clostridium* and *Enterobacteriaceae,* has been traditionally associated with formula fed infants. However, modern infant formulas more closely represent breast milk, shifting the gut microbiota towards beneficial species such as lactobacilli [19,36]. Breast-fed infants are less likely to develop NEC as breast milk contains many protective bioactives [1]. The initial neonatal microbiota consists of facultative anaerobic bacteria such as *Enterobacteriaceae,* enterococci, streptococci and staphylococci, which are present within days of birth [33]. These bacteria consume oxygen providing the reducing conditions required for the growth of obligate anaerobes, typically bifidobacteria, clostridia and *Bacteroides,* appearing one to two weeks later [33,36]. It is well established that the intestinal microbiota has a profound effect on gut health, influencing physiology and metabolism, as well as maturing the infant immune system and protecting against pathogens [19,33]. However, in the preterm infant, the normal succession of bacterial colonisers may be interrupted by the administration of broad-spectrum antibiotics, gut immaturity, acquisition of nosocomial bacteria in the NICU and placement of orogastric or nasogastric feeding tubes, resulting in a more restricted enteric microbiota with delayed colonisation with bifidobacteria and without the individual differences seen in the healthy, term neonate [6,33,37]. The relationship between delayed succession, bacterial overgrowth and NEC is discussed in more detail elsewhere in this chapter.

2. The role of microbes in NEC

The belief bacteria are crucial for the development of NEC stems from a number of clinical and experimental findings. In two studies totalling over 100 infants, Sántulli et al and Schullinger et al were the first to credibly establish bacterial colonisation of the neonatal intestine was a requirement for this disease [38,39]. NEC does not usually occur immediately post-partum but some days later, when feeding has usually commenced and there is ample opportunity for substantial intestinal colonisation. Early-onset NEC occurs in the first week and it is more often seen in term or near term infants with risk factors such as cardiac disease or severe placental insufficiency, whereas in infants of lower gestational age/birth-weight, NEC is delayed until

http://dx.doi.org/10.5772/55039

13-32 days [40,41]. The reason for this difference is not entirely clear, but it may relate to a difference in pathophysiology, with bowel ischaemia being the predominant factor in early-onset NEC and cytokine priming being the predominant factor in late-onset NEC. The case for bacterial colonisation is further strengthened by the absence of NEC in ischaemic, ileal segments of germ-free rats and in infants who are stillborn [42,43].

Regardless of the initiating factors, pathological changes certainly involve bacteria as the intramural gas produced in pneumatosis intestinalis contains hydrogen of bacterial origin [44]. Demonstration of bacteria and bacterial DNA in the intestinal wall of resected segments from NEC infants supports this finding [45,46]. Epidemiological studies also indicate NEC has an infectious origin as it may occur in clusters of related cases which are amenable to infection control measures [47]. Moreover, prevention of NEC has been achieved through the administration of enteral antibiotics [48]. Bacteraemia and endotoxinaemia are frequent complications of NEC but are more likely to be sequelae rather than the actual cause [49,50]. Historically, there have been many proposals put forward regarding the aetiology of NEC (reviewed by Obladen [14]) but two main theories have emerged concerning the infectious component:

Specific pathogen theory

This theory relies on the existence of a hitherto undiscovered, single bacterial pathogen causing intestinal infection in susceptible infants.

Abnormal colonisation theory

Even in health, many members of the enteric microbiota can be considered to have pathogenic potential. When the balance between pathogenic and commensal species shifts in favour of the former, a chain of events is triggered in susceptible infants resulting in NEC.

2.1. Microbes implicated in the aetiology of NEC

Enteric anaerobes

Among the enteric anaerobes, *Clostridium* species are notorious for their proteolytic, saccharolytic, toxin and gas producing activities, making them ideal candidate microorganisms for the specific pathogen theory. Pederson et al emphasised the similarities between neonatal NEC and gas gangrene of the bowel, suggesting that ischaemic lesions were ideal sites for clostridial invasion, the anaerobic conditions of the bowel favouring conversion of the spores to toxin-producing bacteria [51]. Studying the histology of resected intestinal segments from NEC infants led these researchers to conclude *Clostridium perfringens* (*C. welchii*) type A was the most likely cause. Some early experiments on germ-free rats showed injection of *C. perfringens* spores into the intestinal wall induced pneumatosis intestinalis, whereas a variety of other intestinal bacteria did not [52]. Parallels were drawn with pigbel, an acute necrotising enterocolitis common in older children and adults in Papua New Guinea, caused by type C porcine *Clostridium perfringens* [52,53]. These and other findings focused attention on the clostridia for many years. Several investigations indicated *C. perfringens* was more commonly isolated from NEC infants prior to, and at the time of presentation compared to control infants [54–56]. However, negative findings include the long-term study of Dittmar et al where *C. perfrin-*

gens was present in only nine of 41 cases of NEC, with organisms mostly recovered from the peritoneal cavity rather than stool, while Gupta et al did not detect clostridia in any of 23 NEC cases [57,58]. Although it's unlikely *C. perfringens* is the specific pathogen in NEC, intestinal colonisation with this organism was observed to be associated with a more severe form of the disease, a finding supported by Kosloske and Ulrich, and Bjornvad et al in an animal model [45,57,59]. As the oxygen tension of healthy tissue is likely to inhibit growth of clostridia, pre-existing tissue necrosis may be exigent. The hypothesis that clostridial alpha-toxin plays a major role in NEC has never been proven [57].

C. difficile produces two large molecular weight toxins known to cause antibiotic-associated colitis. Somewhat surprisingly, colonisation with this microbe seems not to be a risk factor for NEC, probably because the neonatal bowel is tolerant to *C. difficile* toxins [55,60,61]. *C. butyricum* has been advocated as a cause of NEC but Blakey et al found it was not more common in patients compared to controls [55]. A novel *Clostridium*, designated *C.* 'neonatale' was purported to be the cause of an outbreak of NEC in a Canadian hospital but has not been reported since [62].

Other intestinal anaerobic genera have not been fully investigated, probably due to the difficulty of culturing under strict anaerobic conditions. Despite the prevailing view that non-sporing anaerobes are frequently absent in the intestinal tract of preterm infants, a DNA-based study indicated *Bacteroides* were abundant, and a review of anaerobic bacteraemia in a NICU carried out by Noel et al indicated anaerobic bacteraemia was frequently linked to NEC [63,64]. It is likely that further culture-independent studies will be able to better define the contribution these bacteria make to the pathogenesis of NEC.

Staphylococci

Coagulase negative staphylococci (CoNS) are commonly found in the stools of NEC infants and have been associated with significant disease [65,66]. Hoy et al noted their presence in duodenal aspirates of VLBW infants [10]. The role of staphylococcal delta(δ)-toxin was examined by Scheifele et al and Scheifele and Bjornson, who believed that toxin positive CoNS were enteropathic [67,68]. δ-toxin, a secreted protein with a detergent-like action, caused significant bowel necrosis in infant rats and was cytotoxic for fibroblasts in vitro. Moreover, it could be detected in the stools of infants colonised with δ-toxin producing CoNS [67,68].

We investigated 25 CoNS isolates from the stools of six NEC and six control infants in Dunedin Hospital NICU. A diagnosis of NEC was made on the basis of clinical indications and pneumatosis intestinalis or peritonitis on X-ray as described previously [69]. CoNS were identified using API ID-32 STAPH strips (bioMérieux). PCR primers for the δ-toxin gene were based on sequence data published by Tegmark et al and PCR conditions were as described by McIntosh [70,71]. Cell-free culture supernatants of the CoNS isolates and a δ-toxin producing *S. aureus* control were tested for cell damage (cytopathic effect; CPE) against the small and large intestinal tissue culture cell lines, Caco2 and HT29 [70]. The results, summarised in Table 2, suggest that the δ-toxin gene was frequently present in CoNS isolated from the infants (23 of 25 isolates) but that insufficient toxin was produced to cause a CPE in either of the cell lines tested compared to the *Staphylococcus aureus* control, which induced cell death. Reduced potency of exotoxins is a common feature of CoNS such as *S. epidermidis*, and probably explains their low virulence compared to *S. aureus* [72]. However, this may not always be the case. We found the culture supernatant of a single *S. epidermidis* isolate among 29 CoNS isolated from the skin and nares of University of Otago undergraduate students which could induce a cytopathic effect in the intestinal cell lines (Table 2). The toxic strain was positive for the δ-toxin gene by PCR and Southern hybridisation, although we lacked the specific antibody required to ultimately prove the cytopathic activity was δ-toxin mediated. The δ-toxin theory has been largely dismissed, but our research suggests there may be occasional strains of *S. epidermidis* producing significant amounts of toxin. The findings of Scheifele et al may reflect the dominance of such strains at a particular time in their NICU. There is one instance of a small outbreak of NEC and bacteraemia associated with a δ-toxin-producing methicillin resistant *S. aureus*, supporting the hypothesis that this toxin may contribute to the pathology of NEC providing it is produced in sufficient quantities in vivo [73].

Rejection of the δ-toxin theory does not preclude a role for CoNS *per se*, which are known to express a number of other virulence factors [74]. In addition, preterm infants exhibit deficiencies in immune responses to CoNS, suggesting they may cause more aggressive infections in this group compared to term neonates [75]. Large, relatively stable reservoirs of CoNS have been identified in the faces, ear region, axillae and nares of preterm infants, with smaller, less stable populations elsewhere on the skin, indicating the widespread presence of this group of bacteria and their easy access to the GI tract [76].

Subjects	**NEC infants (n=6)**		**non-NEC infants (n=6)**		**Students (n=19)**	
CoNS isolates tested	**n=15**		**n=10**		**n=29**	
Staphylococcus:	†δ +	‡CPE	δ +	CPE	δ +	CPE
S. epidermidis	11	0	6	0	15	1
Other	3	0	3	0	13	0

†δ + indicates presence of delta-toxin gene

‡CPE: cytopathic effect of CoNS culture supernatant on intestinal cell lines HT29 and Caco2.

Table 2. Presence of delta-toxin gene and cytopathic effect of coagulase-negative staphylococci colonies cultured from the stools of infants with and without necrotising enterocolitis and the skin/nares of university students.

Enterobacteriaceae

The *Enterobacteriaceae* family includes both classical enteric pathogens, such as *Salmonella, Shigella* and diarrhoeagenic *Escherichia coli*, and commensals inhabiting the large intestine. It is the commensals that are common in the enteric microbiota of neonates, including those who develop NEC. Despite their commensal status, these enterobacteria often possess specific virulence factors and are a common cause of extra-intestinal infection. There are early reports of a particular association between *Klebsiella, E. coli* and NEC, with isolation of the same organisms from the blood in some cases [77–79]. A number of subsequent studies have demonstrated their predominance in the faecal microbiota and duodenal aspirates of NEC infants [3,10,58,80]. *Enterobacter cloacae, Klebsiella* spp. and *E. coli* appear to be the most common NEC-associated bacteria overall [3,69,77–79,81]. With the exception of *Cronobacter* (*Enterobacter*) *sakazakii*, which appears to be a special case, many other investigations have not shown a link between particular species or strains and NEC.

Characteristics of *E. cloacae* relevant to the pathogenesis of NEC include resistance to complement-mediated killing (serum resistance), adherence to and invasion of eukaryotic cells in vitro and chelation of iron [69,82]. In *Klebsiella* species, bacterial capsules are responsible for resistance to complement-mediated killing and phagocytosis by polymorphonuclear granulocytes as well as inhibition of macrophages. Differences in virulence between strains are believed to depend on the presence of repetitive sugar sequences in the capsule, which mediate lectin-dependent phagocytosis [83]. Adherence to eukaryotic cells and iron chelation are other virulence factors reported in *Klebsiella* [69,83]. More recently, a cytotoxin has been detected in *K. oxytoca* causing antibiotic-associated haemorrhagic colitis [84]. *E. coli* is notable for its ability to acquire virulence factors which endow it with diarrhoeagenic capacity, but such virulence factors are only occasionally present in isolates from the stools and duodenal aspirates of NEC infants [3,10,58]. *E. coli* cultured from the blood and stools of NEC cases have been shown to pass through epithelial cell monolayers in vitro and highly adherent strains induced NEC-like injury in a weanling rabbit ileal loop model. However, *E. coli* from NEC infants were not shown to be more virulent than those from matched control infants [85,86]. Commensal *Enterobacteriaceae* are not exclusively found in NEC infants, nor are they present in all cases, so they cannot be regarded as the specific pathogen for NEC [3,69,79]. Nevertheless, their frequent occurrence and possession of relevant virulence factors does allow for them to have an important role. Like many other investigators, we have been unable to show *Enterobacteriaceae* cultured from the stools of NEC infants harbour more virulence factors than those without, although the uncertainty regarding the pathogenesis of NEC presents a barrier to discerning essential pathogenic characteristics.

Cronobacter spp. are recognised opportunist pathogens of neonates causing bacteraemia and meningitis as well as being NEC associated. Epidemiological studies have shown powdered infant formula to be the source of the microorganism in many cases although other sources, such as the maternal birth canal are suspected [87,88]. A typical outbreak of *C. sakazakii* associated NEC is described by van Acker et al [89]. Neonates who developed NEC over a two-month period were fed milk formula contaminated with *C. sakazakii*, with a cessation of cases when the formula was removed. *C. sakazakii* is the most common *Cronobacter* species in neonatal infection but does not fulfil the criteria for the single, specific agent of NEC as it is infrequently isolated [87]. The high mortality rate in *C. sakazakii* infection has stimulated research into the virulence of this species, and this is discussed in a later section.

Classical enteric pathogens

Reports citing classical enteric pathogens such as salmonellae and shigellae as causes of NEC or NEC-like conditions are rare [18,90]. Enteric viruses such as norovirus, rotavirus, torovirus, and astrovirus are more frequently implicated. Some investigators consider norovirus to be an emerging pathogen in the NICU, with NEC representing a severe presentation of infection

http://dx.doi.org/10.5772/55039

[91,92]. Human astrovirus was reported by Bagci et al to be the cause of NEC in a subgroup of infants and torovirus was found to be more common in NEC compared to control infants by Lodha et al [93,94]. Rotavirus has been demonstrated in the stools of neonates from day 4 of life and its presence is considered a risk factor for NEC [95]. Echovirus type 22, renamed human parechovirus, is also considered to be an enteric pathogen, although causality has not been fully established [96]. Birenbaum et al detected this virus in an outbreak of diarrhoeal illness in a NICU with some patients exhibiting the clinical signs and symptoms of NEC [97]. Rousset et al noted the presence of coronavirus-like particles in gut tissue samples from NEC infants and proposed that secondary proliferation of anaerobic bacteria occurred in the gut wall following viral damage of the intestinal epithelium [98].

The advent of molecular techniques has facilitated the detection of viruses and it is likely that future investigations will better define the viruses associated with NEC. However, claims that viruses are *the* cause of NEC are not substantiated by the pathology, which strongly supports a role for bacteria. It is more likely that viruses predispose infants to NEC through damage to the epithelium, aiding translocation of the bacteria into the intestinal submucosa. In this regard, both rotavirus and norovirus infections have been shown to lead to epithelial barrier dysfunction through a reduction in sealing tight junctional proteins and an increase in epithelial cell apoptosis [99-101]. Which viruses are involved and how frequently they occur remains open to question as most studies failed to simultaneously investigate the bacteria present, which may have been the invasive organisms causing NEC. It is unlikely that viruses or classical enteric pathogens are the specific pathogens in NEC as they are not universally present. For example, in a comprehensive study of 27 NEC infants, Ullrich et al found common bacterial, viral and parasitic gastrointestinal pathogens were absent in all cases [102]. Gordon et al have proposed viral NEC is a separate disease with a lower mortality rate [13]. However, the difficulty of clinically distinguishing between viral and bacterial NEC, coupled with the likelihood that secondary bacterial invasion occurs, renders this argument more academic than practical.

2.2. Diversity and numbers

It is clear many of the bacteria forming part of the enteric microbiota have pathogenic potential and it has been suggested that when the balance between pathogenic and commensal species shifts in favour of the former, a chain of events is triggered in susceptible infants leading to NEC. A number of studies have sought to investigate this abnormal colonisation theory by identifying and quantifying enteric bacteria at the time of NEC presentation and comparing the results with a control group of healthy infants. However, there is evidence the intestinal ecosystem is altered by inflammation while the microbiota is restored after the inflammatory signal is dissipated [103]. This may be described as a 'chicken and egg' situation; it is unclear whether changes in the microbiota of NEC infants cause the disease or are a result of the inflammation. Of particular value are prospective investigations, as they have the potential to elucidate the microbiota associated with the initiation of NEC

The early, prospective study of Hoy et al was restricted to culturable bacteria, but nevertheless demonstrated considerable quantitative changes in the faecal microbiota preceding both confirmed and suspected episodes of NEC, with a decline in some species up to 72 hours before clinical onset and the emergence of others, particularly *Enterobactericeae* [80]. Most human colonic bacteria are not amenable to culture, so molecular studies constitute a more promising line of enquiry. Techniques are mainly based on the gene encoding the 16S subunit of bacterial ribosomal RNA. This gene has hypervariable regions which are genus- and sometimes species-specific. Sequencing certain hypervariable regions of the 16S rRNA gene and comparing with sequences of known bacteria deposited in databases is now a common and accepted method of identification. Variations of this technique include the use of species-specific fluorescent 16S rDNA probes which bind to bacteria *in situ* (fluorescent *in situ* hybridisation; FISH), and 16S polymerase chain reaction denaturing gel gradient electrophoresis (16S PCR-DGGE) which separates 16S rDNA fragments from the different species present in a mixed community of bacteria.

A recent study encompassing both culture and molecular techniques has strengthened the argument that *Enterobacteriaceae* and staphylococci are important NEC-associated bacteria. In a prospective study, Stewart et al found differences in the gut microbiota of preterm infants who developed NEC or positive blood cultures. Certain Gram-positive genera, *Enterococcus* and *Streptococcus* were more frequent in health while *Enterobacter* and *Staphylococcus* were associated with disease. Moreover, these changes were evident before the onset of clinical symptoms [104]. Mai et al demonstrated the faecal microbiota of preterm infants was more heterogeneous one week before NEC diagnosis, with a low carriage of *Proteobacteria.* In contrast, blooms of *Proteobacteria,* a major phylum including the *Enterobacteriaceae* (*Gammaproteobacteria),* and a decrease in *Firmicutes* subsequently occurred preceding the onset of NEC by at least 72 hours [105]. Other community studies have contrasted the enteric microbiota in infants without NEC with that of NEC infants at the time of presentation. Smith et al analysed tissue samples from infants with fulminant NEC undergoing surgery. Using FISH, communities of bacteria in the excised tissue samples were investigated. *Proteobacteria* were present in most samples, in this instance dominated by *E. coli* and to a lesser extent by *Enterobacter*. Overall composition varied from infant to infant, with some infants showing a high diversity in bacterial species and others a low diversity. Clostridia, present in a few of the neonatal samples, were associated with pneumatosis intestinalis diagnosed histologically but this was considered to be a secondary effect. The study noted the presence of two more unusual bacteria, *Ralstonia* and *Propionibacterium,* in most samples. However, their ubiquitous nature and lack of dominance in the tissues suggests they were not the primary pathogens [106]. Wang et al profiled microbial communities in faecal samples from of 10 NEC infants and 10 non-NEC controls collected at the time of diagnosis. Limited microbial diversity was seen in all the preterm infants with a predominance of *Gammaproteobacteria.* Each infant had a unique microbiota (including twins) and no specific pathogen was implicated. However, differences between NEC and control infants were seen. Microbial community structure in the NEC infants was the least diverse but with a *Proteobacteria* bloom, which was absent in controls, even though the same bacterial species were present. NEC infants had received significantly more antibiotic treatments and it was hypothesised that antibiotics inhibit the bacteria which normally check the growth of *Proteobacteria* [107]. These findings are disputed by Mai et al, who found that overall microbial diversity at the time of diagnosis does not differ between healthy preterm infants and those diagnosed with NEC [105].

A confounding factor is that antibiotic therapy is frequently applied to preterm infants with the possible outcome that the reduced microbial diversity reported to be a feature of NEC could be a consequence of the antibiotic. Tanaka et al demonstrated antibiotic exposure in the pre- or early postnatal period greatly influences the enteric microbiota with arrested growth of beneficial bifidobacteria and overgrowth of *Enterococcus* and higher *Enterobacteriaceae* populations at one month of age [108]. Antibiotic use following preterm rupture of membranes (PROM) may alter the bacterial flora, and the effect of different antibiotic regimens in PROM has been examined with regard to the later occurrence of NEC. The Cochrane review by Kenyon et al found that only beta-lactam antibiotics (including Augmentin) showed an association with later NEC. The relative risk was 4.72 (1.57 – 14.23) compared to placebo, n = 1880. The duration of initial antibiotic treatment in the NICU has also been shown to affect the later occurrence of NEC in extremely low birth-weight (ELBW) infants [109]. Cotten et al used data from 5693 ELBW infants from multiple NICU services to examine the later NEC rate following initial empiric antibiotic use where the cultures proved negative. There were many other risk factors for NEC, some of which were also associated with the duration of antibiotic use, but multivariate analysis allowing for these factors demonstrated that duration of antibiotic use beyond 5 days was associated with an increased risk of NEC [110].

2.3. Significant microorganisms

Despite many attempts, the specific pathogen theory of NEC has not been proven. The strongest candidate organisms, commensal members of the *Enterobacteriaceae,* staphylococci and clostridia are not universally present in NEC infants and may be found in the enteric microbiota of infants without NEC. Clostridia are likely to be secondary invaders rather than primary pathogens. Molecular studies have not uncovered a previously unknown specific pathogen, although uncultured bacteria have been detected in stools of NEC infants [105,111]. The four criteria known as Koch's postulates, designed to establish causality between microbes and disease, are not fulfilled by the existing knowledge of NEC. Gupta et al, who undertook the first comprehensive case/control study of possible microbial causes, were the first to establish this fact [58]. Epidemics of classical enteric pathogens, including diarrhoeagenic *E. coli,* have been associated with NEC from time to time but most cases appear to be associated with normal members of the gut microbiota. *Mycoplasma hominis* and *Ureaplasma urealyticum* are associated with preterm birth but appear not to colonise the human gastrointestinal tract. Using PCR-DGGE, Millar et al were unable to detect these organisms in preterm infants with or without NEC [111]. The claim that enteric viruses cause NEC has not been substantiated although it seems likely that they represent a risk factor. The question of whether NEC infants are colonised by more virulent strains of the same species colonising infants without NEC has not been fully investigated but, as yet, there is little evidence to support such a hypothesis.

The abnormal colonisation theory, with its emphasis on community structure rather than specific organisms, has emerged as the most likely explanation for NEC. Possibly some members of the microbiota contribute to health while others increase the likelihood of NEC, with quantitative changes heralding the onset. Even though they have never been proven to be the causative agents, *Enterobacteriaceae* are commonly found in the gut of infants with NEC and have been isolated from various sites in the body of affected infants [112]. The idea that a bloom of *Proteobacteria* precedes NEC is compatible with existing knowledge and highlights the importance of the Gram-negative *Enterobacteriaceae*. However, this probably does not occur in all cases. For example, Smith et al found Gram-positive bacteria dominated the faecal microbiota of NEC infants whereas a mixed microbiota of Gram-positive and Gram-negative bacteria occurred in the control infants [113]. Further investigation of CoNS is required, as these are a common component of the enteric microbiota in preterm infants and have been implicated in NEC. There is no convincing evidence that intestinal colonisation with enterococci is detrimental to the health of preterm infants. Rather, it may be beneficial, as some strains of *Enterococcus faecalis* have been shown to down-regulate the inflammatory response, modulate innate immune function in intestinal cell lines and to have a protective role in bacterial translocation [85,86,114,115]. In addition to the dominance of certain types of bacteria, NEC aetiology may involve the absence of other bacteria. For example, Blakey et al noted anaerobic *Bacteroides* spp. and lactobacilli were significantly less common in NEC infants compared to controls [55]. The paucity of probiotic bacteria in NEC infants and the phenomenon of microbial interference, where one species of bacteria inhibits another, are discussed elsewhere.

Several studies challenge the long held belief that the foetus is normally devoid of microorganisms and it now seems likely that colonisation begins before birth and can be detrimental. Intrauterine infection is a major cause of prematurity and is associated with adverse neonatal outcomes [116,117]. According to Gonçalves et al, microorganisms gain access to the amniotic cavity and foetus by four main pathways: (1) ascending from the vagina and cervix; (2) transplacental infection; (3) seeding from the peritoneal cavity via the fallopian tubes; (4) accidental introduction during invasive procedures [118]. The ascending pathway is probably the most common route of infection and a variety of microorganisms have been implicated [118]. PCR-based studies, such as that of DiGiulio et al, indicate microbial invasion of the amniotic cavity is common in the setting of preterm, pre-labour rupture of membranes and is underestimated using standard culture techniques [119]. *Mycoplasma* and *Ureaplasma* are the predominant genera in the amniotic cavity whereas NEC associated species are less frequently present [118,119]. Usually clinically silent in the mother, infection of the chorion and amnion are chronic, proinflammatory events believed to have wide-ranging, deleterious effects on the foetus [120]. Several investigations have reported an association between chorioamnionitis and NEC [116, 121–123], although others have failed to show any link [124,125]. A recent meta-analysis of 33 relevant studies revealed a significant association between clinical chorioamnionitis and NEC but there was no association where histological changes alone were the indicator of infection. A threefold increased risk of NEC was seen where chorioamnionitis diagnosed histologically was accompanied by foetal involvement [126]. Additional markers of inflammation, such as umbilical cord polymorphonuclear cell infiltration, *Ureaplasma urealyticum* colonisation and increased cord blood cytokine levels (IL-6, IL-8) have been linked to NEC. However, other studies have been unable to confirm these findings [126].

The mechanisms underlying the relationship between intrauterine infection, the inflammatory pathway and NEC have not been elucidated but animal experimentation indicates intra-amniotic exposure to lipopolysaccharide or *Ureaplasma* induces intestinal inflammation in the foetus resulting in mucosal damage and impaired development of the intestine [127,128]. How closely these findings mirror the human situation remains to be seen. A contrary argument is that the foetal inflammatory response may be protective for neonates because it is already primed to deal with microorganisms interacting with the gut epithelium through the ingestion of microorganisms in amniotic fluid. Histologic chorioamnionitis is not necessarily associated with adverse long-term outcomes and may be protective for late onset sepsis [129,130]. On the other hand, if foetal inflammation is sufficiently damaging, it may predispose the neonate to NEC through impairment of the epithelial barrier. As noted earlier, despite the importance of intrauterine *Ureaplasma* and *Mycoplasma* as a risk factor for NEC, these microorganisms seem not to colonise the intestinal tract [111]. Other bacteria, mainly *E. faecalis*, *S. epidermidis* and *E. coli*, were the predominant species isolated from the meconium of healthy neonates by Jiménez et al who noted that bacteria can be detected in umbilical cord blood, amniotic fluid and foetal membranes in the absence of infection and inflammation [131]. Whether these antenatal gastrointestinal colonisers have a specific role in NEC has not been explored. That NEC occurs some days after birth suggests either additional microorganisms are required or the existing microorganisms need time to multiply in order to reach significant numbers.

2.4. Crossing the epithelial barrier

Structure and function

As previously mentioned, motility patterns in the small bowel are poorly developed in the preterm infant, particularly before 28 weeks gestation, with gastrointestinal transit times ranging from 8-96 hours compared to 4-12 hours in adults [132]. Gastric acid production and enterokinase levels are low in the premature infant, which may limit lipid and protein digestion in the small intestine, and together with lowered intestinal motility may be responsible for bacteria having substrate available for growth for longer periods. In 1990, Carrion and Egan investigated supplementing the feeds of premature infants with hydrochloric acid. The results were promising, but this approach has not been widely adopted, and appears not to have been investigated further [133]. It is postulated that bacterial fermentation of substrate (lactose) present in the infant gut damages the mucosa through the production of gas, which increases intraluminal pressure. The ability of some commensal species to ferment lactose is well known but there seems to be no correlation with NEC [58]. The surface of the gastrointestinal tract must allow entry of molecules that are beneficial to the host while at the same time preventing harmful microbes from crossing the barrier. Piena-Spoel et al observed increased intestinal permeability in human neonates with severe NEC, compared with control babies [134].

The intestinal epithelium from the stomach to the rectum is comprised of a single layer of polarised epithelial cells. The main functions of these cells are to absorb nutrients and also to prevent luminal bacteria and other antigens from crossing the intestinal barrier and entering the bloodstream [88]. Extrinsic barriers including gastric acidity, intestinal peristalsis and the mucus layer limit the access and adhesion of bacteria to the epithelial surface. The mucus layer is an organised extracellular matrix containing inorganic salts, non-specific antimicrobials and specific antimicrobial immunoglobulins, water and large glycoproteins (mucins) [135]. Mucins are produced by goblet cells within the crypts of the intestinal epithelium and released either constitutively or in response to infecting organisms [135]. Intrinsic barriers, which include the selectively permeable epithelial cell plasma membrane and the tight junctions that seal the intracellular spaces, block translocation of bacteria and restrict diffusion of macromolecules. Both these barriers are underdeveloped in the premature infant and this coupled with immaturity of the immune or cellular defense mechanisms may result in bacterial translocation leading to the inflammatory cascade resulting in NEC, even without prior injury of the mucosa. This hypothesis is supported by the fact that mice deficient in Muc2 have been shown both to be susceptible to infection and to develop intestinal inflammation. These mice, as well as having a deficiency in mucus production, had increased leakiness in the gut, which allowed microbes (both commensals and pathogens) to transit the mucosa [136]. Bergstrom et al suggest that the epithelium may be subsequently damaged either as a result of bacteria producing high concentrations of toxic metabolites or, alternatively, the presence of the bacteria stimulates recruitment of large numbers of polymorphonucleocytes to the site of infection resulting in epithelial cell death as neutrophils release cytotoxic mediators to control the infection [136]. The blooms of intestinal *Proteobacteria* seen prior to the onset of NEC in some infants may directly increase their rate of translocation *via* non-specific phagocytic uptake by epithelial cells lining the villi. Indigenous *Enterobacteriaceae* are considered to translocate with the greatest efficiency, *S. epidermidis* with moderate efficiency and obligate anaerobes with the least efficiency [137].

Tight Junctions

Tight junctions and adherens junctions are critical for maintenance of gut permeability and intestinal barrier function [138,139]. Tight junctions form a permeable barrier allowing the passage of fluids and solutes but not the other contents of the intestinal lumen. These junctions are made up of trans-membrane proteins (including occludins, claudins) and junctional adhesion proteins as well as cytoplasmic proteins (zona occludens - ZO-1, ZO-2, ZO-3) [140]. Using an epithelial cell monolayer (Caco2 cells) as in vitro model intestinal barrier, Han et al were able to demonstrate that proinflammatory cytokines interferon -γ, tumor necrosis factor - α and interleukin -1β could affect the expression of occludins and claudins involved in formation of tight junctions [141]. Another study demonstrated that epidermal growth factor prevented the disruption of tight junction proteins in an injury model using Caco-2 monolayers [142]. The importance of occludins and claudins in the formation of functional tight junctions has also been demonstrated in animal models of NEC where a positive correlation between ileal occludin mRNA levels and the progression of ileal injury was noted [143]. Erythropoietin (Epo), a component of human milk, has been suggested to have a physiological role in the developing gut. In vitro studies undertaken by Shiou et al, demonstrated that Epo is able to reverse the effect of IFN - γ and protect ZO-1 expression and barrier function [140]. In a rat model of NEC the same authors demonstrated that oral administration of Epo was able to reduce the incidence of NEC from 45% to 23%. If tight junctions are improperly formed or if

http://dx.doi.org/10.5772/55039

they are damaged as a result of cytokine production in response to bacteria interacting with intestinal epithelial cells then bacteria will be able to translocate into the tissue causing some of the typical symptoms observed in NEC e.g. intramural gas. Reduced tight junction complexes have been associated with chronic inflammation in diseases such as ulcerative colitis and Crohn's disease. In these conditions there are often more bacteria found in association with the epithelium [144].

It is known that signals from the bacteria colonising the gut after birth play a role in maturation of physiological, anatomical and biochemical functions of the intestinal epithelial barrier [145]. Comparisons between conventional and gnotobiotic animals have demonstrated that the microbiota is involved in development, maintenance and repair of the intestinal mucosa [139,145]. As outlined previously, colonisation of the gut in neonates is influenced by gestation, postnatal age, environmental factors such as diet and the rearing environment, and administration of antibiotics. Cilieborg et al conclude that genetically determined gut characteristics (structure, function, immunity) and the time and mode of birth are the most crucial factors in the development of the enteric microbiota, which may be of a beneficial or harmful nature in terms of mucosal integrity [146]. *C. sakazakii* provides a good example of a potentially harmful member of the microbiota in that it is believed to trigger intestinal disease by modulating enterocyte-signalling pathways resulting in cell apoptosis [112]. This pathogen is also notable for its ability to induce the disruption of the tight junctions between enterocytes [147].

Mechanisms

The mechanisms by which classical enteric pathogens cross the intestinal epithelial barrier have been carefully studied as they provide putative targets for the prevention and treatment of infectious diarrhoeal diseases. Adherence is generally the beginning of the colonisation process leading to infection and, for invasive pathogens such as *Salmonella* and the NEC pathogen *C. sakazakii*, adherence is a prerequisite to internalisation in enterocytes. It is generally assumed that NEC-associated bacteria adhere to enterocytes prior to the development of the disease [148,149]. While direct evidence is lacking, animal studies support this contention and, from a theoretical point of view, it could be an essential step [85]. Adherence prevents bacteria being removed by luminal flow allowing them to deliver cytotoxic molecules, endotoxin and other pro-inflammatory substances directly to the epithelium. Features of the preterm intestine previously discussed such as scanty mucous, lack of secretory IgA and delayed colonisation with inhibitory probiotic bacteria certainly provide an opportunity for adherence of commensals to occur. When tested in an in vitro system, we found *Enterobacteriaceae* isolated from stool samples of NEC infants could adhere to both large (HT29) and small (CaCo-2) intestinal cell lines, although most did not adhere to the same extent as the diarrhoeagenic *E. coli* O111 control [69,150]. Such adherent bacteria may act as anchors for the formation of microcolonies on the mucosal surface, facilitating translocation through interactions with the innate immune system.

There is potential for bacterial cytotoxins to assist translocation of bacteria in the gut lumen through induction of enterocyte death. In a pilot study, we investigated 53 *Enterobacteriaceae* colonies cultured from the stools of four infants with NEC (at time of diagnosis) and four infants without NEC for cytotoxin production. The criteria for NEC diagnosis and selection of

NEC –ve infants were as specified by Brooks et al [69]. Cell-free, broth culture supernatants prepared from multiple bacterial colonies per stool sample were tested against a large bowel tissue culture cell line, HT29, as previously described [151]. Cytotoxic supernatants were diluted two-fold and re-tested to obtain the titre. All colonies were identified using API 20E biochemical test strips (bioMérieux). A small minority of the supernatants showed cytotoxic activity (Table 3), but there was no significant difference in their occurrence in NEC versus non-NEC infants or in the amount of toxin produced. Toxin producers were identified as *Serratia marcescens* (both groups), *Klebsiella oxytoca* (NEC positive group), *Escherichia vulneris* and *Klebsiella pneumoniae* ss. *pneumoniae* (NEC negative group). *Serratia marcescens* is known to produce pore-forming toxins, which may explain its cytotoxic activity for HT29 cells [152]. Cytotoxic activity in *Escherichia vulneris* and *Klebsiella pneumoniae* ss. *pneumoniae* is not recorded elsewhere. However, cytotoxin production in some strains of *Klebsiella oxytoca* has recently been described [153].

Infants	**NEC positive (n=4)**		**NEC negative (n=4)**	
Cytotoxin	Positive	Negative	Positive	Negative
Number of isolates	3	30	4	16
Toxin titre range	4–16		8–16	

Table 3. Cytotoxin production in *Enterobacteriaceae* from stool samples of infants with and without necrotising enterocolitis

3. Maturity of the gut and the innate immune response

As described in the previous section, the extrinsic barriers in the premature gut are not fully developed. Goblet cells, found throughout the intestine, are responsible for the secretion of mucus that protects the intestinal lining as well as providing some protections and nutrients for the bacteria that colonise it. There are both secretory mucins (Muc2) and membrane bound mucins (Muc3), which are co-secreted with trefoil factors (TFFs) [139]. The intestine can respond to injury by increasing mucin production. Resident microbes in the gut can also induce an increase in mucin production [154]. Mucins have been implicated in cellular signalling by virtue of the fact that they are able to develop binding sites for lectins, adhesion molecules, cytokines and chemokines. In the immature gut the coverage of mucin is scanty which may facilitate bacterial adherence to the epithelial cells. Paneth cells in the small intestine are able to secrete a wide spectrum of antimicrobial peptides against bacteria, fungi and viruses. Microfold (M) cells in the intestine sample the intestinal environment and deliver antigens to more specialised lymphoid tissue. Their role in disease in the premature neonate is unknown. However, impaired production of both MUC2 and TFF3 has been reported in clinical and experimental cases of NEC [139]. In a rat model of NEC Khailova et al demonstrated that when rats were given a probiotic bacterial strain *Bifidobacterium bifidum* that regulation of the mucin layer was observed with levels of mucin3 and TFF3 similar to those of control animals [139].

The innate immune system of the intestinal epithelium barrier has to be able to distinguish commensal bacteria from pathogens. Pattern recognition receptors on the intestinal epithelial barrier (transmembrane Toll-like receptors and intracellular nucleotide binding oligomerisation domain –like (NOD) receptors) have to be able to recognise microbial ligands (lipopolysaccharide, flagellin, lipotechoic acid, peptidoglycans and formylated peptides) known as microbial-associated molecular patterns (MAMPs). Depending on how the signal is perceived a number of responses can be generated - with commensal bacteria a protective response; with pathogenic bacteria an inflammatory response; or it can be a response that triggers apoptosis [145]. Commensal bacteria can dampen TLR-mediated inflammatory signals. The nuclear factor kappa B (NFκB) transcriptional control pathway has both anti-inflammatory and pro-inflammatory roles dependent on the microbial signal received [145]. Once the MAMP has bound to its respective TLR, the TLR triggers recruitment of the myeloid differentiation primary-response gene 88 (*Myd*88), which then recruits another protein known as IL-1R associated protein kinase. Activation of this gene leads to activation of NFκB and other regulators of gene expression. Along with the expression of inflammatory genes this is the basis of the innate immune response in the gut [155]. Receptors of the innate immune system are expressed on intestinal epithelial cells and also antigen presenting cells such as macrophages and dendritic cells. Discrimination of pathogenic bacteria from commensal bacteria is mediated by the trans membrane TLRs and the intracellular NOD isoforms [155]. The gut associated lymphoid tissue is made up of Peyers Patches, which can be described as mucosal lymph nodes overlaid with M cells. M cells have endocytic organelles that facilitate uptake of antigens from the intestinal lumen. Peyers Patches contain several types of antigen presenting cells such as dendritic cells and B cells. The lamina propria of the gut contains antigen presenting T cells, antibody secreting B cells, T cells and macrophages [156].

The microbiota, mucin and antibacterial products such as defensins and immunoglobulins help protect the host against pathogens. In infants with NEC who have a poorly developed gut with little mucin production and an abnormal microbiota compared to full term healthy infants, the potential for bacteria to cross the intestinal barrier and initiate inflammatory disease is much greater. Once we have a better understanding of the microbial-mucosal signalling components of inflammatory pathways and the regulation of these by commensal bacteria we may be able to find new ways of preventing NEC in premature infants. Alternatively, or as well as, damage to the intestinal mucosa by enteric viruses, harmful members of the gut microbiota, acidic or toxic luminal contents are likely to facilitate translocation. Injury due to hypoxic-ischaemic events in late-onset NEC is generally considered to be transient and unlikely to directly induce translocation. However, there may be subtle effects and when severe, it could be a permissive factor [20].

4. The inflammatory response

The initial step in any infection is the adherence of a microorganism to a host surface. As previously discussed, this binding may trigger a number of host responses such as chemokine and cytokine release, alterations in intracellular signalling pathways and induction of apoptosis. Cytokines play an important role in the regulation of inflammation. In cases of NEC several cytokines have been identified as being associated with the disease. A number of pro-inflammatory cytokines (IL-1β, IL-6, IL-12, IL-18 and TNF-α), an anti-inflammatory cytokine (IL-10) and platelet activating factor (PAF) have been associated with NEC pathogenesis and neonatal sepsis in both infants and in animal models of NEC [157–159].

Pro-inflammatory cytokines can cause increased production of nitric oxide which is known to modulate various physiological processes including inflammation [88,141,]. Nitric oxide is produced from arginine by nitric oxide synthases of which there are three isoforms one of which is inducible (iNOS). This inducible isoform is expressed at high levels during inflammation and is activated by cytokines such as gamma interferon and by bacterial lipopolysaccharide [88,160]. Nitric oxide may cause damage either directly or through its toxic intermediate, $ONOO^-$ resulting in a direct cytopathic effect on the cells (apoptosis) and inhibiting enterocyte proliferation and migration so that the intestinal mucosa cannot repair itself [88]. iNOS knockout mice have been shown to be more susceptible to infection with a number of microorganisms including *Porphyomonas gingivalis* and *Salmonella* [160]. Intestinal iNOS expression increased in the terminal ileum in a rat model of NEC with concurrent enterocyte apoptosis and decreased IL-12 production [161]. IL-12 is involved in bacterial clearance. Surgical specimens from infants with acute NEC have also demonstrated increased levels of iNOS and gamma interferon mRNA [157].

Platelet activating factor (PAF) has also been implicated in cases of NEC. This pro-inflammatory lipid mediator has been associated with intestinal mucosal injury and bowel necrosis in animal models of NEC and neonates with NEC [162,163]. A two-step enzymatic process is used to produce PAF [163]. Experimental animal model research has suggested that both PAF and intestinal bacteria are required to cause NEC as PAF alone cannot induce experimental NEC in a rodent model in the absence of the intestinal microflora [164,165]. PAF is released in response to hypoxia, infection or local injury and Soliman et al hypothesise that this then results in up-regulation of TLR4 in the intestinal epithelium allowing excessive bacterial activation of the intestinal inflammatory response [163]. Another group has also demonstrated that when PAF degrading enzyme is given in association with enteral feeding in a rat model of NEC that initiation of NEC is prevented [166].

IL-10 plays a protective role in the pathogenesis of NEC. Using wild type and IL-10 knockout mice Emami et al have demonstrated that in IL-10 deficient mice there is more evidence of epithelial apoptosis and dissociation of tight junctions compared to wild type animals [159]. In addition, when IL-10 knockout mouse pups were treated with IL-10 or phosphate buffered saline, pups given IL-10 had a greater rate of survival than the PBS treated pups and improved intestinal villus architecture. IL-10 can suppress the secretion of pro-inflammatory cytokines such as IL-2, TNF-α and gamma interferon. This cytokine is found in human breast milk and has been postulated to be one of the protective factors preventing the development of NEC. In addition, IL-10 can suppress expression of iNOS at the mucosal level in macrophages [167]. As described above, high levels of iNOS have been associated with cases of NEC. Lee and Chau have demonstrated that the enzyme heme-oxygenase -1 is induced by IL-10 and that this enzyme is required to mediate the action of IL-10 both in vitro and in vivo. When an HO inhibitor was given to mice, IL-10 mediated protection against LPS-induced septic shock was decreased [167]. IL-10 protection appears to be the result of down regulation of iNOS expression leading to less damage of the intestinal surface. However, if levels of HO-1 are reduced or absent IL-10 is not able to control iNOS expression. Further evidence for the role of NO in NEC has been provided by Ford et al who examined levels of inflammatory cytokines and NO in samples of intestine obtained from infants undergoing surgical resection for NEC and who demonstrated that NO was produced in large amounts by enterocytes in the intestinal wall leading to apoptosis of enterocytes in apical villi through peroxynitrite formation [157].

4.1. Signaling pathways

One of the newer approaches to understanding the pathology of NEC has been at a molecular level and examines the relationship between the intestinal epithelium and commensal bacteria. This research has identified a class of bacterial receptors known as Toll-like receptors (TLRs), in particular TLR 4, whose ability to respond to bacteria associated with the intestinal epithelium may in part explain why some premature infants are susceptible to NEC. More than ten TLRs have so far been identified in humans [168]. These receptors form part of the innate immune response and interact with different components of bacteria and viruses. TLR4, for example, is known to be the receptor for bacterial lipopolysaccharide. As NEC has often been shown to develop after gut colonisation with Gram-negative strains of bacteria, a putative role for TLR4 in the pathogenesis of this disease has been suggested. Mice with mutations in TLR4 or lacking TLR4 do not develop NEC [24,165]. Activation of enterocyte TLR4 leads to increased death of cells in the intestine through the mechanism of apoptosis [169]. TLR4 activation results in stimulation of IL-1R kinase via adaptor molecules MyD88 and MD2 resulting in activation through NFκB and up-regulation of pro-inflammatory cytokines [24]. Gribar et al have demonstrated that TLR4 expression is higher during gestation in the mouse and falls off shortly before birth [170]. They have also postulated a link between TLR4 levels and TLR9 levels in the pathogenesis of NEC. TLR9 recognises bacterial DNA as opposed to LPS recognised by TLR4. TLR4 levels are increased in the bowel of infants with NEC compared to control bowel samples [24]. In a mouse model of NEC, Leaphart et al demonstrated that physiological stressors such as hypoxia and LPS associated with the development of NEC sensitise the epithelium to LPS through the up-regulation of TLR4 and that if animals had a mutation in TLR4 the severity of NEC was reduced due to increased healing capacity of the epithelium [24]. Thus the effect of TLR4 appears to be two-fold by promoting damage to the small intestine through up-regulation of inflammatory cytokines and in reducing mucosal repair. As reported in the last section, there is also a known relationship between TLR4 up-regulation and PAF, one of the molecules implicated in the pathogenesis of NEC.

The relationship between TLR4 and TLR 9 and the signalling from both these receptors has an important role to play in the development of NEC [170]. In cases of NEC, in both humans and mice, increased TLR4 and decreased TLR9 expression was measured. TLR9 recognises CpG motifs of bacterial DNA. Bacterial DNA differs from human DNA in that is enriched with CpG motifs and is largely unmethylated [170]. Using a murine model of NEC, Gibrar et al demonstrated that NEC occurs when there is increased TLR4 and decreased TLR9 expression in developing intestinal mucosa. Furthermore, they were able to show that activation of TLR9 with CpG-DNA inhibited TLR4 mediated signalling in enterocytes. The mechanism of inhibition was dependent upon the inhibitory signalling molecule IL-1R kinase. When CpG-DNA was administered to newborn mice the incidence of experimental NEC was significantly reduced. Other studies have also implicated TLR2 in the pathogenesis of NEC. TLR2 mRNA expression was increased along with TLR4 mRNA and activated NFκB in a neonatal rat model of NEC 48 hours prior to lesions being identified histologically [171,172]. TLR2 mediates host response to Gram-positive bacteria and yeasts through the NFκB pathway [173].

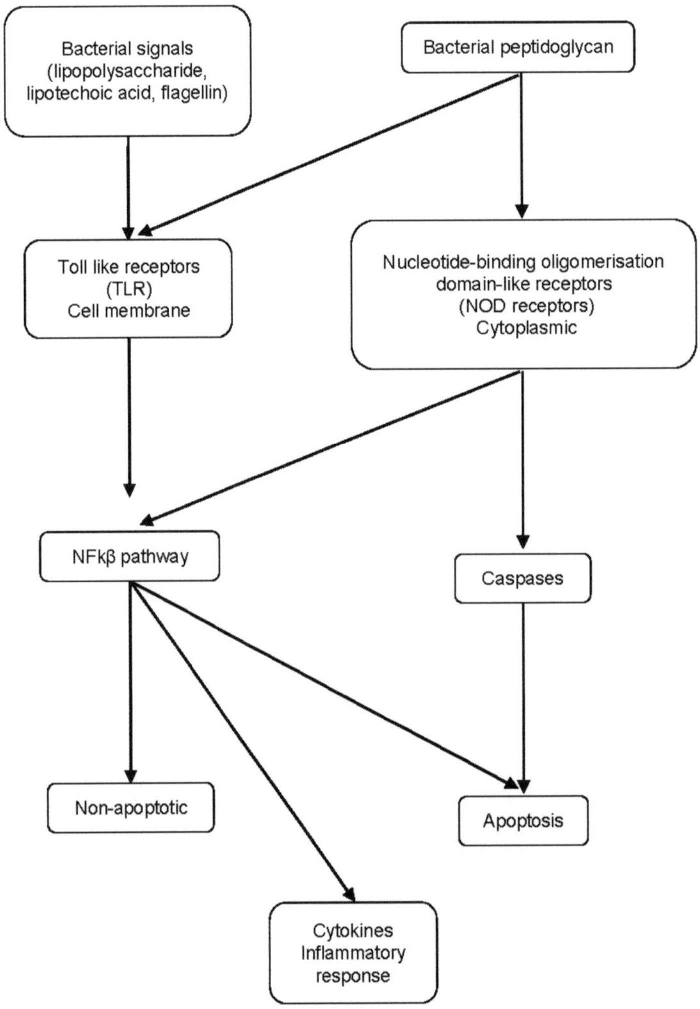

Figure 1. Effects of microbial stimulation on cellular outputs. Toll-like receptors (TLR) and nucleotide-binding oligomerisation domain-like (NOD) receptors recognise patterns of bacterial signals. The outcome of this interaction is variable depending on the commensal or pathogenic status of the bacteria.

Signalling pathways of the innate immune system therefore play an important role in the development of NEC. Understanding of the interactions in this system may lead to the development of new therapeutic treatments for NEC e.g. probiotics with known effects on signalling pathways, anti-inflammatory molecules.

4.2. Cell damage

When pieces of bowel are removed during surgery for NEC and examined histologically, a large number of apoptotic nuclei signifying programmed cell death are observed in the tissues [157]. Studies using an animal model of NEC have demonstrated that apoptosis occurs prior to gross histological damage. When apoptosis was prevented using caspase inhibitors, the development of NEC was significantly reduced [174]. Also, the neonatal pathogen *C. sakazakii* is known to induce apoptosis in enterocytes. As the predominant anatomic lesion of NEC is coagulative or ischaemic necrosis, the contribution of apoptosis requires some explanation [2]. Necrosis is a term currently used by cell biologists for non-apoptotic, accidental cell death and by pathologists to denote the presence of dead tissue or cells regardless of how they have died. In the absence of efficient phagocytosis, apoptotic bodies may lose their integrity and proceed to secondary or apoptotic necrosis. Thus the presence of necrosis indicates cell death has occurred, but does not necessarily indicate how [175].

5. Hypothetical model of NEC

NEC is a complex disease influenced by several risk factors that may act alone and together. The innate immune system appears to play a large role in the establishment of NEC. We propose that in the preterm infant susceptible to NEC, scanty mucus production allows interaction between commensal bacteria and TLR triggering the innate immune response leading to loosening of intercellular tight junctions, enterocyte apoptosis and necrosis, resulting in translocation of bacteria (Figure 2a). Additional factors may also increase translocation, including infection with enteric viruses, presence of microbial cytotoxins or other toxic substances, and a bloom of certain bacteria in the gut lumen causing increased phagocytic uptake by enterocytes. In comparison, the intestinal epithelium of the healthy term neonate secretes adequate mucus, trapping enteric bacteria in the upper layers. In addition, the presence of sIgA and other antimicrobial substance inhibit bacterial colonisation of enterocytes, and any commensal bacteria that do adhere are recognised as not harmful, dampening TLR-mediated inflammatory signals (Figure 2b). In essence, a pivotal event in the development of NEC may be whether the innate immune system of the preterm infant intestine views bacteria reaching the enterocyte surface as friend or foe.

6. Probiotics

Microbial succession ensures that the intestines of healthy neonates are readily colonised with probiotic bacteria such as *Bifidobacterium* and *Lactobacillus*. In contrast, colonisation with these bacteria is delayed in preterm infants [6]. Probiotic bacteria are avirulent, generally of human origin, and purported to have a number of beneficial effects. They are used both prophylactically and as a treatment for certain infections but claims they can colonise the bowel are more controversial, probably because this depends on the specific probiotic. Enteric probiotics may reduce the incidence and severity of diarrhoea due to enteric pathogens through competitive inhibition and/or production of antimicrobial substances. They have been shown to attenuate nitric oxide production, increase antioxidant activities, improve the mucosal barrier, upregulate anti-inflammatory and downregulate pro-inflammatory responses [6-8,176]. Additional probiotic effects, such as regulation of apoptosis and prevention of intestinal injury by *C. sakazakii* have been demonstrated in animal models of NEC [6]. All of these effects are relevant to the prevention of NEC and suggest that probiotics are the ideal, low-cost intervention for preterm and low birth-weight infants. The main difficulty in assessing the efficacy of probiotics for the prevention of NEC is that different bacterial species or strains with different probiotic effects are used in each study, so that the optimum probiotic for NEC, and the biological characteristics that it should possess, have not been well defined.

Trials of probiotics in preterm infants have had varying results. Those reporting a reduction in NEC have often employed *Bifidobacterium*, a dominant genus in the intestines of healthy infants, with or without other probiotic genera [177]. Efficacy in a rat model of NEC has also been demonstrated [139]. Administration of *Bifidobacterium* together with *Lactobacillus* is known to promote the growth of indigenous lactic acid bacteria through the production of short-chain fatty acids [178]. Administration of *Lactobacillus* alone does not appear to prevent NEC and Deshpande et al caution against its use [179]. In the NICU at Dunedin Hospital, Infloran, a probiotic mix of *Bifidobacterium infantis* and *Lactobacillus acidophilus*, is prescribed for infants <1500 g. It has performed well in trials, reducing the incidence of NEC by more than 50% [8]. A recent meta-analysis demonstrated that prophylactic probiotic therapy reduced the incidence of NEC by 30% overall, confirming the significant benefits of supplementation [179]. The risk that in critically ill neonates, or those with compromised gut integrity, probiotics may translocate into the bloodstream has been considered and this is an area requiring further investigation [178,180]. Nevertheless, probiotics are regarded as a promising approach for the prevention of neonatal NEC [7,8].

Cario et al demonstrated that TLR -2 was able to control mucosal inflammation in both in vivo and in vitro models by preserving TJ associated barrier assembly against stress-induced damage via MyD88. When colitis was induced in wild type mice using dextran sodium sulphate followed by treatment with a TLR-2 agonist, clinical signs of colitis were abrogated in all animals when compared to mice which didn't undergo treatment [181]. The probiotic *Bifidobactrium bifidum* was shown to up-regulate expression of TLR-2 in the ileum in a rat model of NEC and this was associated with significantly reduced epithelial apoptosis [139].

Whether probiotic therapy in preterm infants should include supplementation with prebiotics is open to question. Prebiotics promoting the growth of bifidobacteria and lactobacilli are naturally present as oligosaccharides in human milk [8]. The few existing trials of prebiotics in preterm infant have indicated an increase in stool counts of bifidobacteria and lactobacilli occurs. However, until more data is available, routine feed supplementation with prebiotics or synbiotics (probiotic, prebiotic mixtures) is not recommended [6].

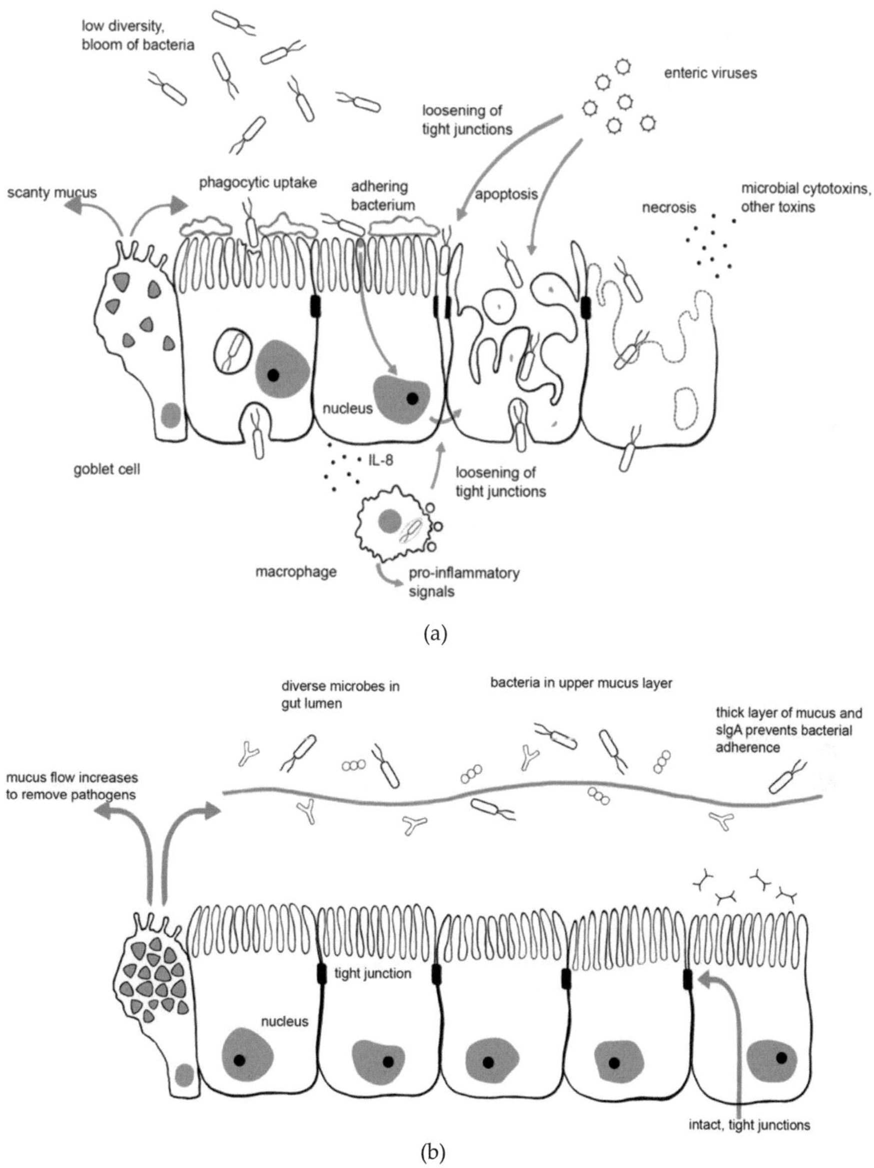

Figure 2. a) Progression of events leading to necrotising enterocolitis in the preterm infant. A bloom of bacteria due to low intestinal motility increases phagocytic uptake. Scanty mucus and reduced antimicrobial factors allow bacteria to adhere to enterocytes, activating NFKB via TRL leading to enterocyte apoptosis, necrosis and loosening of tight junctions. Bacterial translocation may be increased by presence of enteric viruses or microbial and other toxins. b) Intestinal epithelium of the healthy, term neonate. Diversity of enteric microbiota and normal gut motility prevent a bloom of one type of bacteria. Thick mucus, sIgA and other antimicrobial factors inhibit bacterial adherence.

7. Future directions

An article rather pessimistically entitled 'Necrotizing enterocolitis – 150 years of fruitless search for the cause' was published in 2011 [14]. We believe the search has been fruitful and a fuller picture of NEC is now beginning to emerge. NEC is a far more complex disease than early researchers anticipated, involving intrinsic gastrointestinal barriers, the innate immune response, signalling pathways and bacterial colonisation patterns. It seems likely that in individual cases of NEC there will be differences in both the aetiology and pathogenesis. Research into this disease will always be hampered by the fragility and vulnerability of the patients and ethical considerations, leading to a greater dependence on in vitro and animal model experimentation than is usual. Although necessary, antibiotic therapy is often a confounding factor in NEC research because it may eliminate the microbes that initiated the infection. Prospective studies represent a promising avenue of research especially when combined with DNA or RNA based methods for studying changes in the enteric microbiota, initiation of the inflammatory pathway and cell signalling. Through increasing our understanding of NEC, new targets for intervention will be identified. Further investigation of the mechanisms of action of probiotic bacteria will hopefully identify the ideal probiotic for NEC prevention. There is every reason not to be pessimistic about our ability to treat, and more importantly to prevent, this potentially devastating disease of preterm infants in the future.

Acknowledgements

The authors thank H. Fry and D. McComish for preparation of diagrams.

Author details

Heather J.L. Brooks[1*], Michelle A. McConnell[1] and Roland S. Broadbent[2]

*Address all correspondence to: heather.brooks@otago.ac.nz

1 Department of Microbiology and Immunology, Otago School of Medical Sciences, University of Otago, New Zealand

2 Department of Women and Children's Health, Dunedin School of Medicine, University of Otago, New Zealand

References

[1] Schnabl KL, Van Aerde JE, Thomson AB, Clandinin MT. Necrotizing enterocolitis: a multifactorial disease with no cure. World J Gastroenterol 2008;14:2142–2161.

[2] Hsueh W, De Plaen IG, Caplan MS, Qu X-W, Tan X-D, Gonzalez-Crussi F. Neonatal necrotizing enterocolitis: clinical aspects, experimental models and pathogenesis. World J Pediatr 2007;3:17–29.

[3] Boccia D, Stolfi I, Lana S, Moro ML. Nosocomial necrotizing enterocolitis outbreaks: epidemiology and control measures. Eur J Pediatr 2001;160:385–391.

[4] Noerr B. Part 1. Current controversies in the understanding of necrotizing enterocolitis. Adv Neonatal Care 2003;3:107–120.

[5] Lin PW, Stoll BJ. Necrotising enterocolitis. Lancet 2006;368:1271–1283.

[6] Stenger MR, Reber KM, Giannone PJ, Nankervis CA. Probiotics and prebiotics for the prevention of necrotizing enterocolitis. Curr Infect Dis Rep 2011;13:13–20.

[7] Wu S-F, Caplan M, Lin H-C. Necrotizing enterocolitis: old problems with new hope. Pediatr Neonatol 2012;53:158–163.

[8] Caplan MS. Probiotic and prebiotic supplementation for the prevention of neonatal necrotizing enterocolitis. J Perinatol 2009;29:S2–S6.

[9] Neu J, Walker WA. Necrotizing enterocolitis. N Engl J Med 2011;364:255–264.

[10] Hoy CM, Wood CM, Hawkey PM, Puntis JWL. Duodenal microflora in very-low-birth-weight neonates and relation to necrotizing enterocolitis. J Clin Microbiol 2000;68:4539–4547.

[11] Bell MJ, TernbergJL, Feigin RD, Keating J, Marshall R, et al. Neonatal necrotizing enterocolitis: therapeutic decisions based on clinical staging. Ann Surg 1978;187:1–7.

[12] Kliegman RM, Walsh MC. Neonatal necrotizing enterocolitis: pathogenesis, classification, and spectrum of illness. Curr Probl Pediatr 1987;17:213–288.

[13] Gordon PV, Swanson JR, Attridge JT, Clark R. Emerging trends in acquired neonatal intestinal disease: is it time to abandon Bell's criteria? J Perinatol 2007;27:661–671.

[14] Obladen M. Necrotizing enterocolitis – 150 years of fruitless search for the cause. Neonatology 2009;96:203–210.

[15] Khan A, de Waal K. Pneumoperitoneum in a micropremie: Not always NEC. Case Rep Pediatr 2012;doi:10.1155/2012/295657.

[16] Canioni D, Pauliat S, Gaillard JL, Mougenot JF, Bompard Y, Berche P, et al. Histopathology and microbiology of isolated rectal bleeding in neonates: the so-called 'ecchymotic colitis'. Histopathology 1997;30:472–477.

[17] Carman J, Grünebaum M, Gorenstein A, Katz S, Davidson S. Intussusception in a premature infant simulating necrotising enterocolitis. Z Kinderchir 1987;42:49–51.

[18] Sawardekar KP. Shigellosis caused by *Shigella boydii* in a preterm neonate, masquerading as necrotizing enterocolitis. Pediatr Infect Dis J 2005;24:184–185

[19] Emami CN, Petrosyan M, Giuliani S, Williams M, Hunter C, Prasadarao NV, et al. Role of the host defense system and intestinal microbial flora in the pathogenesis of necrotizing enterocolitis. Surg Infect (Larchmt) 2009;10:407–417.

[20] Luo CC, Shih HH, Chiu CH, Lin JN. Translocation of coagulase-negative bacterial staphylococci in rats following intestinal ischemia-reperfusion injury. Biol Neonate 2004;85:151–154.

[21] Zhou W, Zheng XH, Rong X, Huang LG. Establishment and evaluation of three necrotizing enterocolitis models in premature rats. Mol Med Report 2011;4:1333–1338.

[22] Kosloske AM. Epidemiology of necrotizing enterocolitis. Acta Paediatr Suppl 1994;396:2–7.

[23] Young CM, Kingma SD, Neu J. Ischemia-reperfusion and neonatal intestinal injury. J Pediatr 2011;158(Suppl 2):e25–28.

[24] Leaphart CL, Cavallo J, Gribar SC, Cetin S, Li J, Branca MF, Dubowski TD, et al. A critical role for TLR4 in the pathogenesis of necrotizing enterocolitis by modulating intestinal injury and repair. J Immunol 2007;179:4808–4820.

[25] Mohamed A, Shah PS. Transfusion associated necrotizing enterocolitis: a meta-analysis of observational data. Pediatrics 2012;129:529–540.

[26] Paul DA, Mackley A, Novitsky A, Zhao Y, Brooks A, Locke RG. Increased odds of necrotizing enterocolitis after transfusion of red blood cells in premature infants. Pediatrics 2011;127:635–641.

[27] Singh R, Visintainer PF, Frantz ID 3rd, Shah BL, Meyer KM, Favila SA, et al. Association of necrotizing enterocolitis with anemia and packed red blood cell transfusions in preterm infants. J Perinatol 2011;31:176–182.

[28] El-Dib M, Narang S, Lee E, Massaro AN, Aly H. Red blood cell transfusion, feeding and necrotizing enterocolitis in preterm infants. J Perinatol 2011;31:183–187.

[29] Josephson CD, Wesolowski A, Bao G, Sola-Visner MC, Dudell G, Castillejo MI, et al. Do red cell transfusions increase the risk of necrotizing enterocolitis in premature infants? J Pediatr 2010;157:972–978.

[30] Mally P, Golombek SG, Mishra R, Nigam S, Mohandas K, Depalhma H, et al. Association of necrotizing enterocolitis with elective packed red blood cell transfusions in stable, growing, premature neonates. Am J Perinatol 2006;23:451–458.

[31] Blau J, Calo JM, Dozor D, Sutton M, Alpan G, La Gamma EF. Transfusion-related acute gut injury: necrotizing enterocolitis in very low birth weight neonates after packed red blood cell transfusion. J Pediatr 2011;158:403–409.

[32] Krimmel GA, Baker R, Yanowitz TD. Blood transfusion alters the superior mesenteric artery blood flow velocity response to feeding in premature infants. Am J Perinatol 2009;26:99–105.

[33] Sherman MP. New concepts of microbial translocation in the neonatal intestine: mechanisms and prevention. Clin Perinatol 2010;37:565–579.

[34] Cheu HW, Brown DR, Rowe MI. Breath hydrogen excretion as a screening test for the early diagnosis of necrotizing enterocolitis. Am J Dis Child 1989;143:156–159.

[35] Treszl A, Tulassay T, Vasarhelyi B. Genetic basis for necrotizing enterocolitis: risk factors and their relations to genetic polymorphisms. Front Biosci 2006;11:570–580.

[36] Marques TM, Wall R, Ross RP, Fitzgerald GF, Ryan CA, Stanton C. Programming infant gut microbiota: influence of dietary and environmental factors. Curr Opin Biotechnol 2010;21:149–156.

[37] Schwiertz A, Gruhl B, Löbnitz M, Michel P, Radke M, Blaut M. Development of the intestinal bacterial composition in hospitalized preterm infants in comparison with breast-fed, full-term infants. Pediatr Res 2003;54:393–399.

[38] Sántulli TV, Schullinger JN, Heird WC, Gongaware RD, Wigger J, Barlow B, et al. Acute necrotizing enterocolitis in infancy: a review of 64 cases. Pediatrics 1975;55:376–387.

[39] Schullinger JN, Mollitt DL, Vinocur CD, Sántulli TV, Driscoll JM Jr. Neonatal necrotizing enterocolitis: survival, management and complications: a 25-year study. Am J Dis Child 1981;135:612–614.

[40] Grosfeld JL, Cheu H, Schlatter M, West KW, Rescorla FJ. Changing trends in necrotizing enterocolitis. Experience with 302 cases in two decades. Ann Surg 1991;214:300–306.

[41] Yee WH, Soraisham AS, Shah VS, Aziz K, Yoon W, Lee SK; Canadian Neonatal Network. Incidence and timing of presentation of necrotizing enterocolitis in preterm infants. Pediatrics 2012;129:e298–304.

[42] MacKendrick W, Caplan M. Necrotizing enterocolitis: new thoughts about pathogenesis and potential treatment. Pediatr Clin North Am 1993 40:1047–1059.

[43] Musemeche CA, Kosloske AM, Bartow SA, Umland ET. Comparative effects of ischemia, bacteria, and substrate on the pathogenesis of intestinal necrosis. J Pediatr Surg 1986;21:536–538.

[44] Engel RR, Virnig NL, Hunt CE, Levitt MD. Origin of mural gas in necrotizing enterocolitis. Pediatr Res 1973;7:292.

[45] Kosloske AM, Ulrich JA. A bacteriologic basis for the clinical presentations of necrotizing enterocolitis. J Pediatr Surg 1980;15:558–564.

[46] Bucher BT, McDuffie LA, Nurmohammad S, Tarr PI, Warner BB, Hamvas A, et al. Bacterial DNA content in the intestinal wall from infants with necrotizing enterocolitis. J Peditric Surgery 2011;46:1029–1033.

[47] Book LS, Overall JC, Herbst JJ, Britt MR, Epstein B, Jung AL. Clustering of necrotizing enterocolitis: interruption by infection control measures. N Engl J Med 1977;297:984–986.

[48] Bury RG, Tudehope D. Enteral antibiotics for preventing necrotizing enterocolitis in low birthweight or preterm infants. Cochrane Database Syst Rev 2001;1:CD000405.

[49] Palmer SR, Biffin A, Gamsu HR. Outcome of neonatal necrotizing enterocolitis: results of the BAPM/CDSC surveillance study, 1981–84. Arch Dis Child 1989;64:388–394.

[50] Scheifele DW, Olsen E, Fussell S, Pendray M. Spontaneous endotoxinemia in premature infants: correlations with oral feeding and bowel dysfunction. J Pediatr Gastroenterol Nutr 1985;4:67–74.

[51] Pedersen PV, Hansen FH, Halveg AB, Christiansen ED, Justesen T, Høgh P. Necrotising enterocolitis of the newborn – is it gas-gangrene of the bowel? Lancet 1976;2:715–716.

[52] Yale CE, Balish E, Wu JP. The bacterial etiology of pneumatosis cystoides intestinalis. Arch Surg 1974;109:89–94.

[53] Lawrence GW, Lehmann D, Anian G, Coakley CA, Saleu G, Barker MJ, Davis MW. Impact of active immunisation against enteritis necroticans in Papua New Guinea. Lancet 1990;336:1165–1167.

[54] Yu VY, Joseph R, Bajuk B, Orgill A, Astbury J. Necrotizing enerocolitis in very low birthweight infants: a four-year experience. Aust Paediatr J 1984;20:29–33.

[55] Blakey JL, Lubitz L, Campbell NT, Gillam GL, Bishop RF, Barnes GL. Enteric colonization in sporadic neonatal necrotizing enterocolitis. J Pediatr Gastroenterol Nutr 1985;4:591–595.

[56] de la Cochetière MF, Piloquet H, des Robert C, Darmaun D, Glamiche JP, Roze JC. Early intestinal bacterial colonization and necrotizing enterocolitis in premature infants: the putative role of *Clostridium*. Pediatr Res 2004;56:366–370.

[57] Dittmar E, Beyer P, Fischer D, Schäfer V, Schoepe H, Bauer K, et al. Necrotizing enterocolitis of the neonate with *Clostridium perfringens*: diagnosis, clinical course, and role of alpha toxin. Eur J Pediatr 2008;167:891–895.

[58] Gupta S, Morris JG, Panigrahi P, Nataro JP, Glass RI. Endemic necrotizing enterocolitis: lack of association with a specific infectious agent. Pediatr Infect Dis 1994;13:728–734.

[59] Bjornvad CR, Thymann T, Deutz NE, Burrin DG, Jensen SK, Jensen BB, et al. Enteral feeding induces diet-dependent mucosal dysfunction, bacterial proliferation, and necrotizing enterocolitis in preterm pigs on parenteral nutrition. Am J Physiol Gastrointest Liver Physiol 2008;295:G1092–1103.

[60] Lishman AH, Al Jumaili IJ, Elshibly E, Hey E, Record CO. *Clostridium difficile* isolation in neonates in a special care unit. Lack of correlation with necrotizing enterocolitis. Scand J Gastroenterol 1984;19:441–444.

[61] el-Mohandes AE, Keiser JF, Refat M, Jackson BJ. Prevalence and toxigenicity of *Clostridium difficile* isolates in fecal microflora of preterm infants in the intensive care nursery. Biol Neonate 1993;63:225–229.

[62] Alfa MJ, Robson D, Davi M, Bernard K, Van Caeseele P, Harding GK. An outbreak of necrotizing enterocolitis associated with a novel clostridium species in a neonatal intensive care unit. Clin Infect Dis 2002;35:S101–105.

[63] Chang JY, Shin SM, Chun J, Lee JH, Seo JK. Pyrosequencing-based molecular monitoring of the intestinal bacterial colonization in preterm infants. J Pediatr Gastroenterol Nutr 2011;53:512–519.

[64] Noel GJ, Laufer DA, Edelson PJ. Anaerobic bacteremia in a neonatal intensive care unit: an eighteen-year experience. Pediatr Infect Dis J 1988;7:858–862.

[65] Mollitt DL, Tepas JJ, Talbert JL. The role of coagulase-negative *Staphylococcus* in neonatal necrotizing enterocolitis. J Pediatr Surg 1988;23:60–63.

[66] Coates EW, Karlowicz MG, Croitoru DP, Buescher ES. Distinctive distribution of pathogens associated with peritonitis in neonates with focal intestinal perforation compared with necrotizing enterocolitis. Pediatrics 2005;116:241–246.

[67] Scheifele DW, Bjornson GL, Dyer RA, Dimmick JE. Delta-like toxin produced by coagulase-negative staphylococci is associated with neonatal necrotizing enterocolitis. Infect Immun 1987;55:2268–2273.

[68] Scheifele DW, Bjornson GL. Delta toxin activity in coagulase-negative staphylococci from the bowels of neonates. J Clin Microbiol 1988;26:279–282.

[69] Brooks HJ, McConnell MA,, Corbett J, Buchan GS, Fitzpatrick CE, Broadbent RS. Potential prophylactic value of bovine colostrum in necrotizing enterocolitis in neonates: an in vitro study on bacterial attachment, antibody levels and cytokine production. FEMS Immunol Med Microbiol 2006;48:347–354.

[70] McIntosh SM. The role of coagulase negative staphylococcal delta toxin in necrotizing enterocolitis. MSc thesis, University of Otago, Dunedin, New Zealand.

[71] Tegmark K, Morfeldt E, Arvidson S. Regulation of agr-dependent virulence genes in *Staphylococcus aureus* by RNAIII from coagulase-negative staphylococci. J Bacteriol. 1998;180:3181–3186.

[72] Cheung GY, Rigby K, Wang R, Queck SY, Braughton KR, Whitney AR, et al. *Staphylococcus epidermidis* strategies to avoid killing by human neutrophils. PLoS Pathog 2010;6:e1001133.

[73] Overturf GD, Sherman MP, Scheifele DW, Wong LC. Neonatal necrotizing enterocolitis associated with delta toxin-producing methicillin-resistant *Staphylococcus aureus*. Pediatr Infect Dis J 1990;9:88–91.

[74] Otto M. Virulence factors of the coagulase-negative staphylococci. Front Biosci 2004;9:841–863.

[75] Strunk T, Richmond P, Simmer K, Currie A, Levy O, Burgner D. Neonatal immune responses to coagulase-negative staphylococci. Curr Opin Infect Dis 2007;20:370–375.

[76] Eastwick K, Leeming JP, Bennett D, Millar MR. Reservoirs of coagulase negative staphylococci in preterm infants. Arch Dis Child 1996;74:F99–F104.

[77] Wilson SE, Woolley MM. Primary necrotizing enterocolitis in infants. Arch Surg 1969;99:563–566.

[78] Reid WD, Shannon MP. Necrotizing enterocolitis--a medical approach to treatment. Can Med Assoc J 1973;108:573–576.

[79] Frantz ID 3rd, L'heureux P, Engel RR, Hunt CE. Necrotizing enterocolitis. J Pediatr 1975;86:259–263.

[80] Hoy C, Millar MR, MacKay P, Godwin PGR, Langdale V, Levene MI. Quantitative changes in faecal microflora preceding necrotizing enterocolitis in premature neonates. Arch Dis Child 1990;65:1057–1059.

[81] Krediet TG, van Lelyveld N, Vijlbrief DC, Brouwers HA, Kramer WL, Fleer A, et al. Microbiological factors associated with neonatal necrotizing enterocolitis:protective effect of early antibiotic treatment. Acta Paediatr 2003;92:1180–1182.

[82] Keller R, Pedroso MZ, Ritchmann R, Silva RM. Occurrence of virulence-associated properties in *Enterobacter cloacae*. Infect Immun 1998;66:645–649.

[83] Podschun R, Ullmann U. *Klebsiella* spp. as nosocomial pathogens: epidemiology, taxonomy, typing methods, and pathogenicity factors. Clin Microbiol Rev 1998;11:589–603.

[84] Hoffmann KM, Deutschmann A, Weitzer C, Joainig M, Zechner E, Högenauer C, et al. Antibiotic-associated hemorrhagic colitis caused by cytotoxin-producing *Klebsiella oxytoca*. Pediatrics 2010;125:e960–963.

[85] Panigrahi P, Gupta S, Gewolb IH, Morris JG Jr. Occurrence of necrotizing enterocolitis may be dependent on patterns of bacterial adherence and intestinal colonization:

studies in Caco-2 tissue culture and weanling rabbit models. Pediatr Res 1994;36:115–121.

[86] Panigrahi P, Bamford P, Horvath K, Morris JG Jr, Gewolb IH. *Escherichia coli* transcytosis in a Caco-2 cell model: implications in neonatal necrotizing enterocolitis. Pediatr Res 1996;40:415–421.

[87] Yan QQ, Condell O, Power K, Butler F, Tall BD, Fanning S. *Cronobacter* species (formerly known as *Enterobacter sakazakii*) in powdered infant formula: a review of our current understanding of the biology of this bacterium. J Appl Microbiol 2012;113:1–15.

[88] Petrosyan M, Guner YS, Williams M, Grishin A, Ford HR. Current concepts regarding the pathogenesis of necrotizing enterocolitis. Pediatr Surg Int 2009;25:309–318.

[89] van Acker J, de Smet F, Muyldermans G, Bougatef A, Naessens A, Lauwers S. Outbreak of necrotizing enterocolitis associated with *Enterobacter sakazakii* in powdered milk formula. J Clin Microbiol 2001;39:293–297.

[90] Stein H, Beck J, Solomon A, Schmaman A. Gastroenteritis with necrotizing enterocolitis in premature babies. Br Med J 1972;2:616–619.

[91] Tzialla C, Civardi E, Borghesi A, Sarasini A, Baldanti F, Stronati M. Emerging viral infections in neonatal intensive care unit. J Matern Fetal Neonatal Med 2011;24 Suppl 1:156–158.

[92] Turcios-Ruiz RM, Axelrod P, St John K, Bullitt E, Donahue J, Robinson N, et al. Outbreak of necrotizing enterocolitis caused by norovirus in a neonatal intensive care unit. J Pediatr 2008;153:339–344.

[93] Bagci S, Eis-Hübinger AM, Franz AR, Bierbaum G, Heep A, Schildgen O, et al. Detection of astrovirus in premature infants with necrotizing enterocolitis. Pediatr Infect Dis J 2008;27:347–350.

[94] Lodha A, de Silva N, Petric M, Moore AM. Human torovirus: a new virus associated with neonatal necrotizing enterocolitis. Acta Paediatr 2005;94:1085–1088.

[95] De Villiers FP, Driessen M. Clinical neonatal rotavirus infection: association with necrotising enterocolitis. S Afr Med J 2012;102:620–624.

[96] Harvala H, Simmonds P. Human parechoviruses: biology, epidemiology and clinical significance. J Clin Virol 2009;45:1-9.

[97] Birenbaum E, Handsher R, Kuint J, Dagan R, Raichman B, Mendelson E, et al. Echovirus type 22 outbreak associated with gastro-intestinal disease in aneonatal intensive care unit. Am J Perinatol 1997;14:469–473.

[98] Rousset S, Moscovici O, Lebon P, Barbet JP, Helardot P, Macé B, et al. Intestinal lesions containing coronavirus-like particles in neonatal necrotizing enterocolitis: an ultrastructural analysis. Pediatrics 1984;73:218–224.

[99] Bhowmick R, Halder UC, Chattopadhyay S, Chanda S, Nandi S, Bagchi P, et al. Rotaviral enterotoxin nonstructural protein 4 targets mitochondria for activation of apoptosis during infection. J Biol Chem 2012 doi:10.1074/jbc.M112.369595.

[100] Dickman KG, Hempson SJ, Anderson J, Lippe S, Zhao L, Burakoff R, et al. Rotavirus alters paracellular permeability and energy metabolism in Caco-2 cells. Am J Physiol Gastrointest Liver Physiol 2000;279:G757–766.

[101] Troeger H, Loddenkemper C, Schneider T, Schreier E, Epple HJ, Zeitz M, et al. Structural and functional changes of the duodenum in human norovirus infection. Gut 2009;58:1070–1077.

[102] Ullrich T, Tang YW, Correa H, Garzon SA, Maheshwari A, Hill M, et al. Absence of gastrointestinal pathogens in ileum tissue resected for necrotizing enterocolitis. Pediatr Infect Dis J 2012;31:413–414.

[103] Lupp C, Robertson ML, Wickham ME, Sekirov I, Champion OL, Gaynor EC, et al. Host-mediated inflammation disrupts the intestinal microbiota and promotes the overgrowth of Enterobacteriaceae. Cell Host Microbe 2007;2:119–129.

[104] Stewart C, Marrs E, Magorrian S, Nelson A, Lanyon C, Perry J, et al. The preterm gut microbiota: changes associated with necrotising enterocolitis and infection. Acta Paediatr 2012;doi: 10.1111/j.1651-2227.2012.02801.x.

[105] Mai V, Young CM, Ukhanova M, Wang X, Sun Y, Casella G, et al. Fecal microbiota in premature infants prior to necrotizing enterocolitis. PLoS One 2011;6:e20647.

[106] Smith B, Bodé S, Petersen BL, Jensen TK, Pipper C, Kloppenborg J, et al. Community analysis of bacteria colonizing intestinal tissue of neonates with necrotizing enterocolitis. BMC Microbiol 2011;11:73.

[107] Wang Y, Hoenig JD, Malin KJ, Qamar S, Petrof EO, Sun J, et al. 16S rRNA gene-based analysis of fecal microbiota from preterm infants with and without necrotizing enterocolitis. ISME J 2009;3:944–954.

[108] Tanaka S, Kobayashi T, Songjinda P, Tateyama A, Tsubouchi M, Kiyohara C, et al. Influence of antibiotic exposure in the early postnatal period on the development of intestinal microbiota. FEMS Immunol Med Microbiol 2009;56:80–87.

[109] Kenyon S, Boulvain M, Neilson JP. Antibiotics for preterm rupture of membranes. Cochrane Database Syst Rev 2010;8:CD001058.

[110] Cotten CM, Taylor S, Stoll B, Goldberg RN, Hansen NI, Sánchez PJ, et al; NICHD Neonatal Research Network. Prolonged duration of initial empirical antibiotic treatment is associated with increased rates of necrotizing enterocolitis and death for extremely low birth weight infants. Pediatrics 2009;123:58–66.

[111] Millar MR, Linton CJ, Cade A, Glancy D, Hall M, Jalal H. Application of 16S rRNA gene PCR to study bowel flora of preterm infants with and without necrotizing enterocolitis. J Clin Microbiol 1996;34:2506–2510.

[112] Hunter CJ, Upperman JS, Ford HR, Camerini V. Understanding the susceptibility of the premature infant to necrotizing enterocolitis (NEC). Pediatr Res 2008;63:117–123.

[113] Smith B, Bodé S, Skov TH, Mirsepasi H, Greisen G, Krogfelt KA. Investigation of the early intestinal microflora in premature infants with/without necrotizing enterocolitis using two different methods. Pediatr Res 2012;71:115–120.

[114] Are A, Aronsson L, Wang S, Greicius G, Lee YK, Gustafsson J-Å, et al. *Enterococcus faecalis* from newborn babies regulate endogenous PPARg activity and IL-10 levels in colonic epithelial cells. PNAS 2008;105:1943–1948.

[115] Wang S, Ng LH, Chow WL, Lee YK. Infant intestinal *Enterococcus faecalis* down-regulates inflammatory responses in human intestinal cell lines. World J Gastroenterol 2008;14:1067–1076.

[116] Aziz N, Cheng YW, Caughey AB. Neonatal outcomes in the setting of preterm premature rupture of membranes complicated by chorioamnionitis. J Matern Fetal Neonatal Med 2009;22:780–784.

[117] Reiman M, Kujari H, Ekholm E, Lapinleimu H, Lehtonen L, Haataja L, PIPARI Study Group. Interleukin-6 polymorphism is associated with chorioamnionitis and neonatal infections in preterm infants. J Pediatr 2008;153:19–24.

[118] Gonçalves LF, Chaiworapongsa T, Romero R. Intrauterine infection and prematurity. Ment Retard Dev Disabil Res Rev 2002;8:3–13.

[119] DiGiulio DB, Romero R, Kusanovic JP, Gómez R, Kim CJ, Seok KS, et al. Prevalence and diversity of microbes in the amniotic fluid, the fetal inflammatory response, and pregnancy outcome in women with preterm pre-labor rupture of membranes. Am J Reprod Immunol 2010;64:38–57.

[120] Gantert M, Been JV, Gavilanes AW, Garnier Y, Zimmermann LJ, Kramer BW. Chorioamnionitis: a multiorgan disease of the fetus? J Perinatol 2010;30:S21–30.

[121] Been JV, Rours IG, Kornelisse RF, Lima Passos V, Kramer BW, Schneider TA, et al. Histologic chorioamnionitis, fetal involvement, and antenatal steroids: effects on neonatal outcome in preterm infants. Am J Obstet Gynecol 2009;201:587 e1–8.

[122] Elimian A, Verma U, Beneck D, Cipriano R, Visintainer P, Tejani N. Histologic chorioamnionitis, antenatal steroids, and perinatal outcomes. Obstet Gynecol 2000;96:333–336.

[123] Lau J, Magee F, Qiu Z, Houbé J, Von Dadelszen P, Lee SK. Chorioamnionitis with a fetal inflammatory response is associated with higher neonatal mortality, morbidity,

and resource use than chorioamnionitis displaying a maternal inflammatory response only. Am J Obstet Gynecol 2005;193:708–713.

[124] Dempsey E, Chen MF, Kokottis T, Vallerand D, Usher R. Outcome of neonates less than 30 weeks gestation with histologic chorioamnionitis. Am J Perinatol 2005;22:155–159.

[125] Soraisham AS, Singhal N, McMillan DD, Sauve RS, Lee SK; Canadian Neonatal Network. A multicenter study on the clinical outcome of chorioamnionitis in preterm infants. Am J Obstet Gynecol 2009;200:372e1–6.

[126] Been JV, Lievense S, Zimmermann LJ, Kramer BW, Wolfs TG. Chorioamnionitis as a risk factor for necrotizing enterocolitis: a systematic review and meta-analysis. J Pediatr 2012; doi.org/10.1016/j.jpeds.2012.07.012.

[127] Wolfs TG, Buurman WA, Zoer B, Moonen RM, Derikx JP, Thuijls G, et al. Endotoxin induced chorioamnionitis prevents intestinal development during gestation in fetal sheep. PLoS One 2009;4:e5837.

[128] Wolfs TG, Kallapur SG, Polglase GR, Pillow JJ, Nitsos I, Newnham JP, et al. IL-1α mediated chorioamnionitis induces depletion of FoxP3+ cells and ileal inflammation in the ovine fetal gut. PLoS One 2011;6:e18355.

[129] Bersani I, Thomas W, Speer CP. Chorioamnionitis - the good or the evil for neonatal outcome? J Matern Fetal Neonatal Med 2012;25 Suppl 1:12–16.

[130] Hendson L, Russell L, Robertson CM, Liang Y, Chen Y, Abdalla A, et al. Neonatal and neurodevelopmental outcomes of very low birthweight infants with histologic chorioamnionitis. J Pediatr 2011;158:397–402.

[131] Jiménez E, Marín ML, Martín R, Odriozola JM, Olivares M, Xaus J, et al. Is meconium from healthy newborns actually sterile? Res Microbiol 2008;159:187–193.

[132] Blackburn ST. Gastrointestinal and hepatic systems and perinatal nutrition. In: Maternal, Fetal and Neonatal Physiology 2007;447–448 (Saunders Elsevier, St. Louis, Missouri, USA).

[133] Carrion V, Egan EA. Prevention of neonatal necrotizing enterocolitis. J Pediatr Gastroenterol Nutr 1990;11:317–323.

[134] Piena-Spoel M, Albers MJ, ten Kate J, Tibboel D. Intestinal permeability in newborns with necrotising enterocolitis and controls: does the sugar absorption test provide guideline for the time to (re-) introduce enteral nutrition? J Pediatr Surg 2001;36:587–592.

[135] McGuckin MA, Linden SK, Sutton P, Florin TH. Mucin dynamics and enteric pathogens. Nat Rev Microbiol 2011;9:265–278.

[136] Bergstrom KSB, Kissoon-Singh V, Gibson DL, Ma C, Montero M, Sham HP, et al. Muc2 protects against lethal infectious colitis by disassociating pathogenic and commensal bacteria from the colonic mucosa. PLoS Pathog 2010;6:e1000902.

[137] Berg RD. Bacterial translocation from the gastrointestinal tract. Trends Microbiol 1995;3:149–154.

[138] Khailova L, Dvorak K, Arganbright KM, Williams CS, Hapern MD, Dvorak B. Changes in hepatic cell junctions structure during experimental necrotizing enterocolitis: effect of EGF treatment. Pediatr Res 2009;66:140–144.

[139] Khailova L, Mount Patrick SK, Arganbright KM, Halpern MD, Kinouchi T, Dvorak B. *Bifidobacterium bifidum* reduces apoptosis in the intestinal epithelium in necrotizing enterocolitis. Am J Physiol Gastrointest Liver Physiol 2010;299:G1118–1127.

[140] Shiou S-R, Yu Y, Chen S, Ciancio MJ, Petrof EO, Sun J and Claud EC. Erythropoietin protects intestinal epithelial barrier function and lowers the incidence of experimental neonatal necrotizing enterocolitis. J Biol Chem 2011;286:12123–12132.

[141] Han X, Fink MP, Delude RL. Proinflammatory cytokines cause NO-dependent and -independent changes in expression and localization of tight junction proteins in intestinal epithelial cells. Shock 2003;19:229–237.

[142] Sheth P, Seth A, Thangavel M, Basuroy S, Rao RK. Epidermal growth factor prevents acetaldehyde-induced paracellular permeability in Caco-2 cell monolayer. Alcohol Clin Exp Res 2004;28:797–804.

[143] Clark JA, Doelle SM, Halpern MD, Saunders TA, Holubec H, Dvorak K, et al. Intestinal barrier failure during experimental necrotizing enterocolitis: protective effect of EGF treatment. Am J Physiol Gastrointest Liver Physiol 2006;291:G938 –949.

[144] O'Callaghan J, Buttó LF, MacSharry J, Nally K, O'Toole PW 2012. Influence of adhesion and bacteriocin production by *Lactobacillus salivarius* on the intestinal epithelial cell transcriptional response. Appl Environ Microbiol 2012;78:5196–5203.

[145] Sharma R and Tepas JJ 3rd. Microecology, intestinal epithelial barrier and necrotizing enterocolitis. Pediatr Surg Int 2010;26:11–21.

[146] Cilieborg MS, Boye M, Sanglid PT. Bacterial colonization and gut development in preterm neonates. Early Hum Dev 2012;88:S41–S49.

[147] Liu Q, Mittal R, Emami CN, Iversen C, Ford HR, Prasadarao NV. Human Isolates of *Cronobacter sakazakii* bind efficiently to intestinal epithelial cells in vitro to induce monolayer permeability and apoptosis. J Surg Res 2012;176:437–447.

[148] Dai D, Walker WA. Protective nutrients and bacterial colonization in the immature human gut. Adv Pediatr 1999;46:353–382.

[149] Hsueh W, Caplan MS, Qu X-W, Tan X-D, De Plaen IG, Gonzalez-Crussi F. Neonatal necrotizing enterocolitis: clinical considerations and pathogenetic concepts. Pediatr Dev Pathol 2002;6:6–23.

[150] Filipovska-Naumovska E. Study on the aetiology of necrotizing enterocolitis in premature neonates. MSc thesis, University of Otago, Dunedin, New Zealand.

[151] Inder A. Role of bacterial toxins in the aetiology of necrotising enterocolitis. Bachelor of Medical Science thesis, University of Otago, Dunedin, New Zealand.

[152] Hertle R. The family of *Serratia* type pore forming toxins. Curr Protein Pept Sci 2005;6:313–325.

[153] Hoffmann KM, Deutschmann A, Weitzer C, Joainig M, Zechner E, Högenauer C,et al. Antibiotic-associated hemorrhagic colitis caused by cytotoxin-producing *Klebsiella oxytoca*. Pediatrics 2010;125:e960–963.

[154] Neu J, Douglas-Escobar M. Gastrointestinal development: implications for infant feeding. In Nutrition in Pediatrics, ed. Duggan C, Watkins JB and Walker VA, 4th ed. pp. 241–249 (BC Decker Inc., Hamilton, Ontario, Canada).

[155] Sharma R, Young C and Neu J. Molecular modulation of intestinal epithelial barrier: contribution of microbiota. J Biomed Biotechnol 2010;doi:10.1155/2010/305879.

[156] Eberl G. Inducible lymphoid tissues in the adult gut: recapitulation of a fetal developmental pathway? Nat Rev Immunol 2005;5:413–420.

[157] Ford H, Watkins S, Reblock K and Rowe M. The role of inflammatory cytokines and nitric oxide in the pathogenesis of necrotizing enterocolitis. J Pediatr Surg 1997;32:275–282.

[158] Sharma R, Tepas JJ 3rd, Hudak ML, Mollitt DL, Wludyka PS, Teng R-J, et al. Neonatal gut barrier and multiple organ failure: role of endotoxin and proinflammatory cytokines in sepsis and necrotizing enterocolitis. J Pediatr Surg 2007;42:454–461.

[159] Emami CN, Choski N, Wang J, Hunter C, Guner Y, Goth K, et al. Role of interlukin-10 in the pathogenesis of necrotizing enterocolitis. Am J Surg 2012;203:428–435.

[160] Gyurko R, Boustany G, Huang PL, Kantarci A, Van Dyke TE, Genco CA. Mice lacking inducible nitrate oxide synthase demonstrate impared killing of *Porphyromonas gingivalis*. Infect Immun 2003;71:4917–4924.

[161] Nadler EP, Dickinson E, Knisely A, Zhang X-R, Boyle P, Beer-Stolz D, et al. Expression of inducible nitric oxide synthase and interleukin-12 in experimental necrotizing enterocolitis. J Surg Res 2000;92:71–77.

[162] Upperman JS, Camerini V, Lugo B, Yotov I, Sullivan J, Ribin J, Clermont G, et al. Mathermatical modeling in necrotizing enterocolitis - a new look at an ongoing problem. J Pediatr Surg 2007;42:445–453.

[163] Soliman A, Michelson KS, Karahashi H, Lu J, Meng FJ, Qu X, Crother TR, et al. Platelet-activating factor induces TLR4 expression in intestinal epithelial cells: implication for the pathogenesis of necrotizing enterocolitis PLoS One 2010;5:e15044, doi:10.1371/journal.pone.0015044.

[164] Schriffen EJ, Trop M, Schroeder S and Carter EA. Platelet-activating factor induces intestinal necrosis, but not septic shock, in germ-free and specific-pathogen-free rodents. Burns 1991;17:276–278.

[165] Jilling T, Simon D, Lu J, Meng FJ, Li D, Schy R, et al. The roles of bacteria and TLR4 in rat and murine models of necrotizing enterocolitis. J Immunol 2006;177:3273–3282.

[166] Caplan MS, Hedlund E, Adler L, Lickerman M, Hsueh W. The platelet-activating factor receptor antagonist WEB 2170 prevents necrotizing enterocolitis in rats. J Pediatr Gastroenterol Nutr 1997;24:296–301.

[167] Lee TS, and Chau LY. Heme oxygenase-1 mediates the anti-inflammatory effects of interleukin-10 in mice. Nat Med 2002;8:240–246.

[168] Jilling T, Lu J, Caplan MS. Intestinal epithelial cell apoptosis, immunoregulatory molecules, and necrotizing enterocolitis. J Clin Cell Immunol 2012;S3:007. doi 10.4172/2155-9899.

[169] Afrazi A, Sodhi CP, Richardson W, Neal M, Good M, Siggers R, et al. New insights into the pathogenesis and treatment of necrotizing enterocolitis: toll-like receptors and beyond. Pediatr Res 2011;69:183–188.

[170] Gribar SC, Sodhi CP, Richardson WM, Anand RJ, Gittes GK, Branca MF, et al. Reciprocal Expression and signalling of TLR4 and TLR9 in the pathogenesis and treatment of necrotizing enterocolitis. J Immunol 2009;182:636–646.

[171] Le Mandat Schultz A, Bonnard A, Barreau F, Aigrain Y, Pierre-Louis C, Berrebi D, et al. Expression of TLR-2, TLR-4, NOD2 and pNF-κB in a neonatal rat model of necrotizing enterocolitis. PLoS One 2007;2:e1102. doi:10.1371/journal.pone0001102.

[172] Liu Y, Zhu L, Fatheree NY, Liu X, Pacheco SE, Tatevian N, Rhoads JM. Changes in intestinal Toll-like receptors and cytokines precede histological injury in a rat model of necrotizing enterocolitis. Am J Physiol Gastrointest Liver Physiol 2009;297:G442–450.

[173] Arancibia SA, Beltran CJ, Aguirre IM, Silva P, Peralta AL, Malinarich F, et al. Toll-like receptors are key participants in innate immune responses. Biol Res 2007;40:97–112.

[174] Jilling T, Lu J, Jackson M, Caplan MS. Intestinal epithelial apoptosis initiates gross bowel necrosis in an experimental rat model of neonatal necrotizing enterocolitis. Pediatr Res 2004;55:622–629.

[175] Fink SL, Cookson BT. Apoptosis, pyroptosis, and necrosis: mechanistic description of dead and dying eukaryotic cells. Infect Immun 2005;73:1907–1916.

[176] Hickey L, Jacobs SE, Garland SM. Probiotics in neonatology. J Paediatr Child Health 2012;doi:10.1111/j.1440-1754.2012.02508.x.

[177] Caplan MS, Jilling T. Neonatal necrotizing enterocolitis: possible role of probiotic supplementation. J Pediatr Gastroenterol Nutr 2000;30:S18–22.

[178] Deshpande GC, Rao SC, Keil AD, Patole SK. Evidence-based guidelines for use of probiotics in preterm neonates. BMC Med 2011;9;92.doi: 10.1186/1741-7015-9-92.

[179] Deshpande G, Rao S, Patole S, Bulsara M. Updated meta-analysis of probiotics for preventing necrotizing enterocolitis in preterm neonates. Pediatrics 2010;125:921–930.

[180] Morowitz MJ, Poroyko V, Caplan M, Alverdy J, Liu DC. Redefining the role of intestinal microbes in the pathogenesis of necrotizing enterocolitis. Pediatr 2010;125:777–785.

[181] Cario E, Gerken G and Podolsky DK. Toll-like receptor 2 controls mucosal inflammation by regulating epithelial barrier function. Gastroenterology 2007;132:1359–1374.

Chapter 6

Moderate Preterm Children Born at 32-36 Weeks Gestational Age Around 8 Years of Age: Differences Between Children with and Without Identified Developmental and School Problems

Anneloes L. van Baar, Marjanneke de Jong and Marjolein Verhoeven

Additional information is available at the end of the chapter

http://dx.doi.org/10.5772/54623

1. Introduction

Preterm birth rates have been reported as 12% in the United States and 5–8% in Europe, e.g. in The Netherlands [1, 2]. Mortality rates in preterm children decreased considerably in the last decades, especially for the extreme preterm born children < 28 weeks' gestation [3]. However, 80-90% of the preterm children are born between 32 and 37 weeks' gestation: increasing birth rates in this subgroup have been reported for the last decades [4].Therefore, the number of surviving children increases, and morbidity and developmental outcome of these children become more important: for the children and their families, but also for societies. All preterm children are at increased risk for developmental problems, in all domains of development, with a gradient effect that children born earlier are at greater risk [5].

In recent years, more attention has been given to the development of moderate preterm born children. Moderate preterm birth between 32 and 36+6 weeks occurs in 6-9% of all births [1, 2], which implies that many families are affected each year. Moderate preterm birth also constitutes an insult for the still immature brain of the infant. Several studies reported on outcome of moderate preterm children born between 32 through 36+6 weeks.

A review showed that, overall, more school problems, less advanced cognitive functioning, more behavior problems, and a higher prevalence of psychiatric disorders was found in moderate and late preterm born infants, children, and adults compared with their full term peers [6].

Despite the fact that the risk for developmental problems of moderate preterm born children has become increasingly clear, not many systematic and long term follow up monitoring is done as yet. Further study is needed on the processes and factors that may shape the developmental trajectories of moderate preterm born children. Such information needs to provide guidelines to design an adequate monitoring program.

We studied a sample in The Netherlands of 377 moderate preterm born 7-9 year old children, who were not referred for neonatal intensive care treatment. Cognitive and emotional regulation difficulties were found to affect their functioning, as school problems, a slightly lower IQ, attention and behavioral problems appeared when the moderate preterm children were compared with 182 term born children [7]. Lower educational attainment and more specifically attention and learning difficulties, arose as a core problem for these children. The outcome of the children at school age showed that for some children developmental problems already were identified, because of their attendance of schools for special education or need for grade retention. Other behavioral problems or psychopathology, also may already have been identified by school age, through use of regular care facilities by parents or schools.

In this chapter will be presented for how many moderate preterm children at school age diagnoses or worries concerning developmental and learning problems were indicated by their parents or teachers. Next, the subgroups of moderate preterm children with and without such problems will be compared concerning their neonatal characteristics. In addition their functioning at school age will be compared on the measurements used in our study regarding IQ, sustained attention, and behavior problems. This information may elucidate what kind of developmental problems are found among moderate preterm children and what neonatal characteristics may carry a higher risk. In addition, it may clarify if most children identified through our measurements with low IQ or problems with sustained attention or behavioral problems, were already identified by their parents or teachers, in that they already had a diagnosis or a need for school adjustment before we examined them around 8 years of age. These analyses may result in important information for the design of follow up studies or monitoring procedures of moderate preterm children.

2. Methods

2.1. Participants

Selection criteria for the preterm children consisted of: a gestational age at birth of 32 through 36 weeks + 6 days, no dysmaturity (<P10), no NICU admittance needed, no severe congenital malformations, 7-9 years old. The sample was described in detail in an earlier publication [7]. In short, it consisted of 377 children, 52% boys, with a mean gestation of 34.7 (1.2) weeks and a mean birth weight of 2425 (455) grams. The distribution of 32, 33, 34, 35 and 36 completed weeks of gestation in the preterm group consisted of respectively 6%, 11%, 20%, 28% and 36%. Birth weight was below 2500 grams in 56% with two cases below 1500 grams.

2.2. Instruments

All parents completed a background information questionnaire concerning school situation of the index child, family circumstances, life style during pregnancy, and delivery characteristics. Neonatal data of the preterm children were collected from the hospital files. Cognitive abilities of the children were assessed with the Revised Amsterdam Children's Intelligence Test (RAKIT, short version) for 4 to 11 years [26]. The norm score (IQ score) is 100 (SD = 15) and the mean for the subtests is 15 (SD=5). The test has good psychometric characteristics with an internal consistency coefficient of: 92 and a test-retest coefficient of: 85. A correlation of: 81 was found with a Dutch version of the Wechsler intelligence test – revised [8].

To measure sustained selective attention, the Bourdon-Vos test was used [9]. On a page with 33 horizontal rows of 24 small figures made of three, four or five dots, the children are asked to mark the configurations that consist of four dots, as quickly as possible. Time to complete the rows and the total page is recorded and norm scores have been provided. The validity, sensitivity, and reliability of the test have been found acceptable by the Dutch COTAN organisation that checks test characteristics [10].

Both parents and teachers were asked to complete a questionnaire on competences and behavior problems, the Child Behavior Check List (CBCL) or Teacher Report Form (TRF) [11]. The CBCL and TRF are parallel forms with good psychometric qualities. Scoring provides an assessment of total number of problems, as well as separate scores for internalizing and externalizing behavior problems. A T-score of 60 indicates a cut off for children with many behavior problems, as was found for 15% of the norm population. A further division allows separate results for dimensions of anxious/depressed behavior, physical complaints, social problems, thought problems, attention problems and aggressive behavior.

Information on school outcome (i.e. attending a grade appropriate for age, grade retention, or attending a school for special education) was obtained from the parental background questionnaire or the CBCL and TRF questionnaires. School problems were defined as either attending a school for special education, or having repeated a grade in the regular primary school.

Diagnoses or worries related to daily functioning of the children were indicated by parents on the background questionnaire, or in comments to the test leaders who could note such information as particularities of the child. Based upon the information provided in these comments, difficulties in functioning were differentiated into 11 specific problems.

1. 'Health' concerned problems like asthma, diabetes, eczema.
2. 'Senses' reflected need for hearing aids or glasses.
3. 'Motor problems' indicated illness of Perthes, difficulties in sitting.
4. 'Concentration problems' were noted when difficulties with sustained attention were mentioned.
5. 'Learning problems' reflected a developmental delay or use of Remedial Teaching.
6. 'Dyslexia' was mentioned as such.

7. 'Language problems' indicated treatment by a speech therapist, but also problems in reading, spelling or speech.

8. 'ADHD' was mentioned as such.

9. 'Social emotional problems' reflected anxiety, worries concerning sensitivity and it was mentioned as such.

10. 'Autistic Spectrum' was mentioned as problems within the autistic spectrum.

11. 'Behavioral Adjustment problems' indicated adaptation problems and (hyper)-active behavior.

Although for some children more than one problem was indicated, the information was summarized by an experienced health psychologist (ALvB) into one exclusive code that seemed to represent the most important problem for the child: e.g. when a child was attending a school for children with motor problems and both motor problems and concentration problems were indicated, a final code of 'Motor problems' was assigned.

These problems were summarized into three main developmental domains, distinguishing: 1) the somatic domain (difficulties related to chronic health problems, senses of perception, motor functioning), 2) the cognitive domain (attention deficit hyperactivity disorder (ADHD), concentration problems, learning difficulties, dyslexia, and language problems), and 3) the social-emotional domain (diagnoses within the autistic spectrum, and social-emotional difficulties). In addition a separate code was entered for problems appearing in school functioning (need for special education, grade retention).

Finally a separate code was entered to identify the children that either had any school problem, or any other problem in one of the domains, as described above, creating two subgroups of children with or without any problems.

2.3. Procedure

The participating preterm children were born between 1996 and 1998 in one of seven general hospitals in the south of The Netherlands. The preterm children were selected based upon the hospitals' archives. Their addresses were traced and their parents were contacted and asked for participation.

The study was approved by the Committee of Medical Ethics of the St. Elisabeth hospital in Tilburg and by the committees of the other participating hospitals. The parents gave their written informed consent.

3. Statistical analyses

Descriptive information of the groups with and without developmental problems was compared using analyses of variance and chi-square analyses. Group comparisons concerning the different outcome measures were done using multivariate and univariate analyses of variance or crossstabs. All analyses were done with SPSS 20.0.

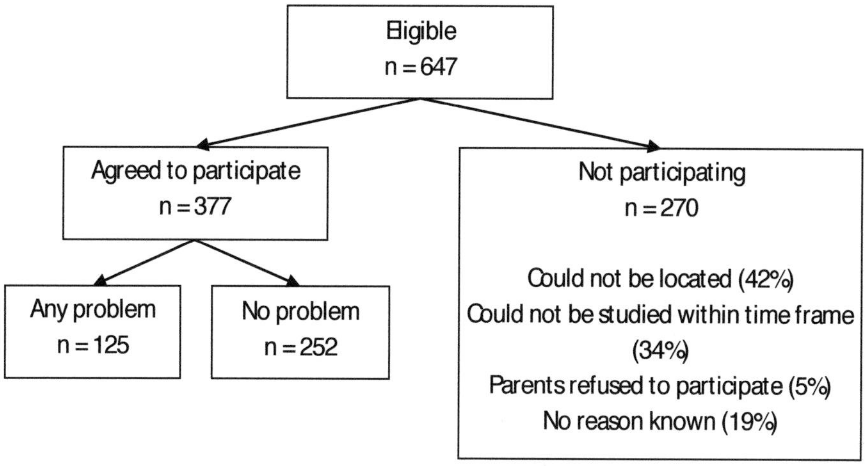

Figure 1. Flow chart of the study design

4. Results

Figure 1 presents the flow chart of the study design. It shows that for 252 children no problems and for 125 children any problem had been indicated by parents or teachers when they entered our study. For 13 out of 87 children (15%) more than one problem had been indicated, e.g. ADHD and behavior problems (coded as ADHD) or motor problems and concentration difficulties (coded as motor problems), but only one code was given.

The amount and kind of developmental problems identified in the moderate preterm children through their school situation and through the diagnoses and worries indicated by parents and teachers are presented in Table 1 per developmental domain and specific kind of problems.

For one third of the moderate preterm children a school or any other developmental problem was found. For 23% of the total group of preterm children a problem in one of the three domains was identified and for 22.6% a school problem was found.

Of the children for whom a specific problem in the somatic, cognitive or social-emotional domain was indicated, 47 (54%) were also found to have a school problem: 22 (25%) of these children attended a special school and 35 (40%) (also) had experienced grade retention. For 40 (46%) of these children no school problems were found.

For 22 (76%) of the children that attended a special school, and for 35 (50%) of the children that had had a grade retention, a specific problem was identified. For 38 (45%) of the children with school problems, no specific problem in one of the domains was indicated.

Forty children, 14% of all preterm children without school problems, were identified with a specific problem in one of the domains.

Domain	Problem	N	% of preterm children
Somatic	Health	16	4.24
	Senses	10	2.65
	Motor functioning	3	0.80
Cognitive	Concentration	8	2.12
	Learning	19	5.04
	Dyslexia	5	1.33
	Language	4	1.06
	ADHD[1]	3	0.80
Social emotional	Social emotional problems	5	1.33
	Autistic spectrum	8	2.12
	Behavioral adjustment	6	1.59
Subtotal		87	23.08
School	Special education	29	7.69
	Grade retention	70	18.57
Subtotal		85	22.55
School or other problem		125	33.2

[1]ADHD = Attention Deficit/Hyperactivity Disorder

Table 1. Identified problems

In Table 2, the background characteristics and neonatal complications are presented for the subgroups with and without any identified developmental problem. In the subgroup of preterm children with any problem (n = 125) significantly more boys were found, chi-square= 11.80, df=1, p=.000.

A marginally significant effect was found regarding the need for oxygen at any time in the neonatal treatment period, which was needed by more children in the group with any problem, chi-square= 3.75, df=1, p=.053. In the total group of preterm children, oxygen was needed by 23% of the children, and for 9% was indicated that they only needed it right after birth. Fifteen children needed oxygen for 3 - 7 days. For the groups with and without problems respectively oxygen only right after birth was needed in 12 (11.3%) versus 16 (7.8%) children, and need for oxygen for 3-7 days in 6 (5.6%) versus 9 (4.4%) children.

No differences between the subgroups with and without any problem were found for other indicators of neonatal complications like gestational age, birth weight, hypoglycaemia, need for phototherapy or the duration of hospital treatment. Distribution of 32, 33, 34, 35 and 36 completed weeks of gestation was for the group with problems respectively 8%, 13%, 23%, 26% and 30%, and for the group without problems 4%, 10%, 21%, 30% and 34%, a non significant difference.

The subgroups did differ in parental education of mothers, in that parents of children with problems were less often highly educated; for mothers chi-square= 7.07, df=2, p=.029; for fathers chi-square= 5.86, df=2, p=.053.

These characteristics of the children and their parents were also compared per domain of development, i.e. somatic, cognitive, or social emotional problems, but this did not show any statistically significant differences.

	Preterm Total group	**No problems N=252**	**Any problem N=125**
Boys, n (%)	197 (52)	116 (46)	81 (65)*
Mean gestation (sd), weeks, range	34.7 (1.2) 32-36	34.8 (1.1) 32-36	34.6 (1.3) 32-36
Mean birth weight (sd), grams, range	2425 (455) 1340-4130	2448 (432) 1340-3564	2380 (497) 1530-4130
Mean days hospital (sd) range	15.7 (10.0) 2-51	15.2 (9.7) 2-49	16.8 (10.5) 2-51
Oxygen needed, n (%)*	71 (22.6)	40 (19.2)	31 (29.2)
Phototherapy, n (%)	162 (43.3)	103 (41)	59 (48)
Hypoglycemia, n (%)	41 (13.2)	30 (14.3)	11 (10.9)
Multiples, n (%)	85 (22.5)	64 (25.4)	21 (16.8)
Mothers education, n (%)*			
Primary level	16 (4.4)	8 (3.3)	8 (6.7)
Secondary level	283 (78.2)	183 (75.9)	100 (82.6)
Tertiary level	63 (17.4)	50 (20.7)	13 (10.8)
Fathers education n (%)*			
Primary level	11(3)	5 (2.1)	6 (5.5)
Secondary level	235 (67)	155(64.9)	80 (72.7)
Tertiary level	103 (29)*	78 (32.8)	25 (22.5)

Note. Analyses of variance and Chi-square analyses comparing the no problem and any problem groups

*p <.05

Table 2. Neonatal and demographic characteristics based upon identified problems

In Table 3 results are presented for the measurements of intelligence and behavioral problems, when the children were around 8 years old. The results are presented for the subgroups with and without any problem in the first two columns, as well as for the subgroups according to main domain of problems in the last three columns. The number of children that actually show a worrisome level of functioning, i.e. that scored at least one standard deviation below the norm IQ score, or above the cut off for a worrisome level of behavior problems, is presented too.

	No problems	**Any problem**	**Somatic domain**	**Cognitive domain**	**Social emotional domain**
	M[1] (sd)[2]	M (sd)	M (sd)	M (sd)	M (sd)
IQ[3]	107 (13.8)	95 (14.6)*	95 (16.0)	91 (16.6)	101 (13.4)
Sustained Attention	6.8 (2.9)	8.1 (2.5)*	7.7 (2.3)	7.7 (2.8)	8.2 (2.8)
CBCL[4] Total – Mothers	50 (9.2)	57 (10.0)*	53 (9.4)	58 (9.6)	65. (8.1)
CBCL Total – Fathers	47 (9.6)	53 (10.3)*	51 (10.4)	55 (9.5)	58 (12.4)
TRF[5] Total – Teachers	50 (8.2)	55 (8.7)*	52 (8.4)	57 (8.2)	62 (8.4)
	N (%)	N (%)	N (%)	N (%)	N (%)
IQ < 85	13 (5.2)	29 (23.6)*	7 (24.1)	13 (33.3)	3 (16.7)
Sustained Attention > 8 decile	93 (37.1)	69 (58.5)*	15 (51.7)	20 (57.1)	11 (64.7)
CBCL Mothers T > 60	39 (16.2)	45 (37.5)*	4 (14.8)	17 (43.6)	14 (73.7)*
CBCL Fathers T > 60	19 (8.3)	26 (25)*	4 (18.1)	11 (33.3)	7 (46.6)
TRF Teachers T > 60	34 (14.7)	38 (34.9)*	6 (23)	18 (48.6)	11 (64.7)*

*Difference between subgroups with or without any problem = p<.01

[1]M = Mean

[2]sd = Standard deviation

[3]IQ = Intelligence Quotient

[4]CBCL = Child Behavior Checklist

[5]TRF = Teacher Report Form

Table 3. Developmental outcome by subgroup based upon identified problems

The subgroups with and without problems differ significantly in all measurements, with lower IQ and more attention and behavior problems for the children whose problems already were identified by parents or teachers (Table 3). This was shown by a multivariate analyses of variance (MANOVA), corrected for sex and maternal education: $F(5,283)=13.62$, $p<.001$, partial eta squared=.194. Univariate analyses of variance showed significant differences for all measurements to the disadvantage of the subgroup with problems.

http://dx.doi.org/10.5772/54623

In addition, more children in the group with identified problems actually showed a worrisome level of functioning on the IQ test, the sustained attention task and the behavior problem questionnaires answered by mothers, fathers and teachers, as chi-square analyses showed significant differences.

A MANOVA corrected for sex and maternal education showed no significant differences between the subgroups with problems in different domains $F(10,112)=1.33$, $p=.225$, partial eta squared=.106. Univariate comparisons did show a difference for the assessment of behavior problems by the mothers, $F(2,82)=9.85$, $p<.001$, and by the teachers, $F(2,77)=7.69$, $p=.001$. These differences indicate that the children with problems in the social emotional domain have more behavior problems than the children who have a main problem in the somatic domain.

As shown by significant chi-square analyses according to mothers and teachers the children who had problems in the somatic domain had less worrisome levels of behavior problems, compared to the children who had a main problem in the cognitive or social-emotional domain.

Only a limited number of children that had a low IQ score (5.2%) or a high problem score on the behavior problem questionnaire (ranging from 8% to 16%) were not identified through the comments of their mothers or teachers (Table 3).

On the sustained attention task, many children in the subgroup without problems (37%) also did show difficulties. Attention problems seem to form a general problem for all moderate preterm children.

5. Discussion

In this chapter was studied for how many of the 377 moderate preterm children examined at school age, developmental problems had already been identified by parents, teachers or school situation. The developmental problems focussed at, appeared through the children's school problems, placement in special schools, earlier diagnoses, or worries concerning daily functioning as indicated by parents and teachers. For a large subgroup, one third of the moderate preterm children studied, school problems or any developmental problem was indeed identified. For 23% of the children a specific problem was indicated. These problems consisted for 10% of cognitive difficulties, for 5% of social-emotional difficulties, and for 8% of difficulties in somatic functioning. Attendance of a special school or grade retention was found in 22% of the preterm children. More than half of the children that were identified with a specific problem, also had a school problem. And, the other way around, for most of the children (76%) that attended a special school, and 50% of the children that had experienced a grade retention, also a specific problem was indicated.

For many children, the difficulties related to school functioning formed their most obvious problem. Beside clear indicators like attendance of a special school, or grade retention, learning problems were also often indicated by parents and teachers and described as difficulties of the child in following the lessons at school. In addition, concentration problems were described in this context. For some children the focus of the description of their problems was put upon behavioral adjustment problems. Few children actually already had a formal diagnosis like ADHD or Dyslexia. A number of children (4%) had mainly health problems, like Asthma, or eczema. This number is not high in view of an estimated prevalence of Asthma in 5-10% of the Dutch population [12].

Therefore it is concluded that most difficulties of moderate preterm children at school age are captured by an indication of school problems. Several other studies also found a greater risk for difficulties in educational attainment. Preschool readiness testing in Florida in the USA showed that at 5 years of age, 13.6% of 22.552 late preterm children (34-37 weeks) versus 11.8% of 164.628 term born children needed special education [13]. In England, risk for not reaching a good level of overall school achievement at age 5 was found to be 12% and 8% higher in respectively moderate preterm and late preterm children compared to term born peers [14]. Children aged 5-7 years and born late preterm in the UK, were also less likely to be successful in school attainment assessments [15]. In a Dutch study, small but significant differences between moderate preterm and term groups were found regarding intelligence, attention and executive functioning at 7 years of age, but no differences appeared for verbal memory, and visuomotor and motor skills [16]. Effects were largest in children with low parental education. For somewhat older moderate and late preterm children in England, aged between 8-11 years, was reported that they more often needed extra educational support at primary school than their term peers, but their IQ scores were similar to those of the full term children [17].

Some other studies also looked at specific learning capacities. Concerning 9-13 year old moderate preterm children in New York city, it was found that they had a 30-50% higher risk of needing special education than full term children. They also had lower adjusted math and English scores than full term children [18]. Also in Scotland, moderate preterm children were found to have a 53% higher risk of special education needs at primary and secondary school (< 19 years of age) compared to term born children [19]. Nomura et al. [20] studied a randomly selected birth cohort (N=1,619) that was followed into adulthood: IQ and learning abilities were measured in childhood and educational attainment was measured in adulthood. Moderate prematurity was associated with lower educational attainment. In adulthood, approximately one-fifth of the cohort had not completed high school, while one-eighth had some college education.

Other developmental problems are also found more frequently within groups of moderate preterm born children. Data from Danish registers of 20.934 children between 2 and 18 years of age, showed that 37 (6,4%) of 581 preterm children, with gestational ages of 34–36 completed weeks, had a clinically verified hyperkinetic disorder [21]. Other studies on behavior problems showed higher scores on all Child Behavior Checklist (CBCL) scales for preschool aged moderate preterm children compared to term born children, particularly for girls [22].

In our study on the moderate preterm children whose problems already had been indicated by parents and teachers at 8 years, we looked also at outcomes of the systematic measures that were used in our follow up study, including the CBCL, IQ tests and measure of attention [7]. The subgroups of children with and without any problem indeed clearly differed on all these measures, as shown in Table 3. A large, 12 point difference in IQ emerged to the disadvantage of the group with problems. In addition all mean total problem scores on the CBCL as assessed by mothers and by fathers and on the TRF reported by the teachers were more than half a standard deviation higher in the group with problems. On the sustained attention task the subgroup with problems also clearly showed more problems. Therefore, the outcome of these measures seems to validate the worries of the parents and teachers and the school situation of most children.

In relation to the specific domain of problems within the subgroup of children with problems only univariate analyses showed subgroup differences. This may partly be the result from statistical power problems. Large differences in some mean scores did appear: e.g. a 10 point difference in IQ to the advantage of the 19 children with mainly social emotional problems, compared to the 39 children with mainly cognitive problems. On a univariate level the children with mainly health problems were found to have less behavior problems as assessed by their mothers and teachers.

A limitation of this study is that the information regarding earlier diagnoses or worries of parents and teachers concerning the children's development was acquired through rather indirect comments. A more systematic way of measurement, using a specific interview or questionnaire, might have revealed more, or other worries of parents and teachers in greater detail. Nevertheless it seemed important to study this indirect information in order to check what kind of difficulties worried parent and teachers, and if unexpected problems would arise. No such unexpected problems were found, and it is concluded that the general protocol used in the follow up study, that focused upon cognitive capacities, attention and behavior problems, actually reflected the worries of the parents and teachers and the problems of the children.

Another limitation of this study was that the data on neonatal complications had to be collected retrospectively from the hospital files. Nowadays, this information is collected digitally, which may improve systematic reporting. Nevertheless, our findings concerning neonatal complications are similar to other reports, e.g. our sample showed hypoglycemia in 13% which compares to the 16% recently reported by Gouyon et al. [23].

In respect to neonatal outcomes, it has been found that in general infants born at 35 to 36+6 weeks (also indicated as late preterm birth) have more medical problems compared to full-term infants [24]. In the current study, neonatal characteristics and complications of the groups with and without problems were also compared. Regarding neonatal complications, a small effect was found indicating that the number of children who had needed oxygen was higher in the subgroup with problems. It could be that these early problems in oxygen supply contributed to less optimal brain development which probably has contributed to the developmental problems of these children. Alternatively, other subtle underlying difficulties may have resulted in the premature birth in itself, or in difficulties adapting to extra uterine life (e.g. need for oxygen), which also caused problems in other areas. No other neonatal complications, like hypoglycaemia or need for phototherapy, systematically differed between the two subgroups. Although a trend could be seen that somewhat more children of a younger gestational age were in the subgroup with developmental problems, this was not a statistically significant effect

An important finding of this study may be that, despite a clear difference between the subgroups with and without problems in the sustained attention task, still many children in the subgroup withóut identified problems had worrisome scores on this task. Attention and concentration problems seem to form a core problem in functioning of moderate preterm children. Other studies also found difficulties in attention capacities of moderate preterm children [6, 16]. Sustained selective attention difficulties have already been found to partially mediate the relation between premature birth and developmental outcome [25].

With regard to characteristics of the children, male sex was more frequently seen in the subgroup of moderate preterm children with problems. Many studies have reported higher risk for preterm boys. Adverse neurodevelopmental outcomes, including moderate to severe Cerebral Palsy, mental and psychomotor developmental indices lower than two standard deviations below the norm, were significantly more likely in extremely low birth weight boys than in girls [5]. In Scotland moderate preterm born boys were found to show a more than two times higher risk of special education needs [19]. Possibly boys are more susceptible for neonatal complications that may affect their brain development. Boys are also more often born preterm than girls, as a 7.2% excess of males was reported for white singleton preterm births and this effect was roughly constant for 20-37 weeks' gestation [26]. Further research on the influence of sex hormones on brain development, starting in the fetal period, and more extensive study on perinatal risk factors in relation to sex of the children, is indicated.

In addition, caretaking processes may differ between boys and girls. Girls may be more sensitive to socialization and stimulation efforts, which may also contribute to differences in developmental outcome, especially in groups at risk. Such processes may also affect development and reinforce or buffer the influence of risk factors.

Another difference found between the subgroups with and without developmental problems concerned parental education. A relationship between developmental outcome and parental education, with more problems in children of lower educated parents, has been reported more frequently. In the study by Cserjesi et al. [16], for instance, small but significant differences between moderate preterm and term groups regarding intelligence, attention and executive functioning were largest in children with low parental education. The relationship with parental education may come about through caretaking and education processes. Parental education however also reflects potentially important genetic and hereditary influences. Further research regarding genetic processes in preterm children is therefore indicated too.

In the group without problems only a limited number of children that had low IQ's or high behavior problem scores were not identified, either through grade retention, need for a special school or explicitly indicated worries of their parents or teachers. An important finding is that many children showed difficulties in the sustained attention task, also in the group without problems. This may indicate that development of attention processes is a sensitive area for all moderate preterm children and further study in this regard is necessary. We did not find many children who had an explicit diagnosis of ADHD, despite the difficulties in attention of many children. Others also found many with attention difficulties, but not with a diagnosis of ADHD, among adolescents born with very low birth weight [27]. Therefore the difficulties in attention skills may be specific for children born with perinatal risk. Further study into specific characteristics of attention processes in relation to perinatal risk factors needs to be done, preferably already at a young age.

Although it is clear that relatively more very preterm children are affected by developmental problems than moderate preterm children, as reported in the literature [5], many moderate preterm children do show serious difficulties. Therefore, it is important to identify such problems as soon as possible, in order to start preventive activities or treatments. Monitoring of development of moderate preterm children in regular follow up programs is necessary. Follow up should be done at younger ages than school age. A systematic follow up procedure should start already in infancy and at toddler age in order to reduce the consequences wherever possible. Development should be followed in all domains. Especially more extensive monitoring should be done of attention development, as most moderate preterm children are found to suffer from difficulties with sustained attention.

Acknowledgements

We thank all the parents and children for their participation. The study was conducted in cooperation between Tilburg university, Elisabeth hospital (J. Bruinenberg) and TweeSteden hospital (J. Bonenkamp) in Tilburg, the Catharina hospital (G. Couturier) in Eindhoven, St Anna hospital (B. van den Boezem) in Geldrop, Elkerliek hospital (E. Brouwer and N. Vaessens) in Helmond, Jeroen Bosch Hospital (C. Jacobs and L. Dekkers) in 's Hertogenbosch, Oosterschelde hospital (A. van der Hoop and J. Bauer) in Goes and Christina van Baalen, Eline Beeren, Anouk de Bruijn, Petra Cobussen, Karin Dekkers, Cathalijn Donders, Ilonka van den Heuvel, Petra de Knecht, Anita Rademakers, Elke van Rijsewijk, Kim Seerden, Yasemin Seref, Malou Smits, Marjolein Volaart, Marijke de Wit.

Author details

Anneloes L. van Baar*, Marjanneke de Jong and Marjolein Verhoeven

*Address all correspondence to: A.L.vanBaar@uu.nl

Department of Child and Adolescent Studies, Utrecht University, Utrecht, the Netherlands

References

[1] Martin JA, Hamilton BE, Ventura SJ, Osterman MJK, Kirmeyer S, Mathews TJ, Wilson EC. Births: final data for 2009. Natl Vital Stat Rep. 2011;60:1-70.

[2] Stichting Perinatale Registratie Nederland. Perinatale zorg in Nederland 2008. Utrecht: Stichting Perinatale Registratie Nederland; 2011.

[3] De Kleine MJK, Den Ouden AL, Kollée LAA, Ilsen A, Van Wassenaer AG, Brand R, Verloove-Vanhorick SP. Lower mortality but higher neonatal morbidity over a decade in very preterm infants. Paediatr Perinat Epidemiol. 2007;21:15–25.

[4] Raju TNK. Epidemiology of late preterm (near-term) births. Clin Perinatol. 2006;33:751-63.

[5] Saigal S, Doyle LW. An overview of mortality and sequelae of preterm birth from infancy to adulthood. Lancet. 2008;371:261-9.

[6] De Jong M, Verhoeven M, Van Baar AL. School outcome, cognitive functioning, and behaviour problems in moderate and late preterm children and adults: A review. Semin Fetal Neonat M. 2012:17;163-9.

[7] Van Baar AL, Vermaas J, Knots E, de Kleine MJK, Soons P. Functioning at School Age of Moderately Preterm Children Born at 32 to 36 Weeks' Gestational Age. Pediatrics. 2009;124:251-7.

[8] Bleichrodt N, Drenth PJD, Zaal JN Resing WCM. RAKIT Handleiding bij de Revisie Amsterdamse Kinder Intelligentie Test. Lisse, The Netherlands: Swets & Zeitlinger; 1987.

[9] Vos P. Handleiding Bourdon-Vos test, 3e herziene uitgave. Lisse: Swets Test Publishers; 1998.

[10] Evers A, van Vliet-Mulder JC, Groot CJ. Documentatie van tests en testresearch in Nederland Deel I Testbeschrijvingen. Assen: Van Gorcum; 2000.

[11] Achenbach TM, Rescorla LA. Manual for the ASEBA school-age forms & profiles. Burlington, VT: University of Vermont, Research Center for Children, Youth & Families; 2001.

[12] Bindels PJE, Van der Wouden JC, Ponsioen BP, Brand PLP, Salomé PL, Van Hensbergen W, Van Hasselt PA, Steenkamer TA, Grol MH. NHG-Standaard Astma bij kinderen (Tweede herziening). Huisarts en Wetenschap. 2006;49:557-72.

[13] Morse SB, Zheng H, Tang Y, Roth J. Early school-age outcomes of late preterm infants. Pediatrics. 2009;123:e622-9.

[14] Quigley MA, Poulsen G, Boyle E, Wolke D, Field D, Alfirevic Z, Kurinczuk JJ. Early term and late preterm birth are associated with poorer school performance at age 5 years: a cohort study. Arch Dis Child Fetal Neonatal Ed. 2012;97:F167-73.

[15] Peacock PJ, Henderson J, Odd D, Emond A. Early school attainment in late-preterm infants. Arch Dis Child. 2012;97:118-20.

[16] Cserjesi R, Van Braeckel KN, Timmerman M, Butcher PR, Kerstjens JM, Reijneveld SA, Bouma A, Bos AF, Geuze RH. Patterns of functioning and predictive factors in children born moderately preterm or at term. Dev Med Child Neurol. 2012;54:710-5.

http://dx.doi.org/10.5772/54623

[17] Odd DE, Emond A, Whitelaw A. Long-term cognitive outcomes of infants born moderately and late preterm. Dev Med Child Neurol. 2012:54;704-9.

[18] Lipkind HS, Slopen ME, Pfeiffer MR, McVeigh KH. School-age outcomes of late preterm infants in New York City. Am J Obstet Gynecol, 2012;206:222.e1-6.

[19] MacKay DF, Smith GCS, Dobbie R, Pell JP. Gestational age at delivery and special educational need: retrospective cohort study of 407,503 schoolchildren. PLoS Medicine. 2010;7:e1000289.

[20] Nomura Y, Halperin JM, Newcorn JH, Davey C, Fifer WP, Savitz DA, Brooks-Gunn J. The risk for impaired learning-related abilities in childhood and educational attainment among adults born near-term. J Pediatr Psychol. 2009;34:406-18.

[21] Linnet KM, Wisborg K, Agerbo E, Secher NJ, Thomsen PH, Henriksen TB. Gestational age, birth weight, and the risk of hyperkinetic disorder. Arch Dis Child. 2006;91:655–60.

[22] Potijk MR, De Winter AF, Bos AF, Kerstjens JM, Reijneveld SA. Higher rates of behavioural and emotional problems at preschool age in children born moderately preterm. Arch Dis Child. 2012;97:112-7.

[23] Gouyon JB, Iacobelli S, Ferdynus C, Bonsante F. Neonatal problems of late and moderate preterm infants. Semin Fetal Neonat M. 2012;17:146-52.

[24] Wang ML, Dorer DJ, Fleming MP, Catlin EA. Clinical outcomes of near-term infants. Pediatrics. 2004;114:372-6

[25] Bul KCM, Van Baar AL. Behavior problems in relation to sustained selective attention skills of moderately preterm children. J Dev Phys Disabil 2012;24:111–23.

[26] Cooperstock M, Campbell J. Excess males in preterm birth: interactions with gestational age, race, and multiple birth. Obstet Gynecol. 1996;88:189-93.

[27] Indredavik, M, Vik T, Heyerdahl S, Kulseng S, Brubakk AM. Psychiatric symptoms in low birth weight adolescents, assessed by screening questionnaires. Eur Child Adolesc Psychiatry. 2005;14:226–36.